Handbook of
Transcranial Doppler

MW00838181

Springer

New York
Berlin
Heidelberg
Barcelona
Budapest
Hong Kong
London
Milan
Paris
Santa Clara
Singapore
Tokyo

Handbook of Transcranial Doppler

John P. McCartney, R.V.T.

Technical Vice President, DWL Electronic Systems, Inc., Santa Clara, CA

Kathleen M. Thomas-Lukes, R.N., M.N.

Clinical Safety Specialist, Department of Safety and Development, Amgen, Inc., Thousand Oaks, CA

Camilo R. Gomez, M.D.

Associate Professor, Department of Neurology, and Director, Comprehensive Stroke Center, University of Alabama at Birmingham, Birmingham, AL

With 88 Illustrations

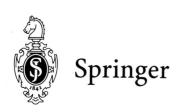

Springer

John P. McCartney, R.V.T.
Technical Vice President
DWL Electronic Systems Inc.
Santa Clara, CA 95051, USA
formerly:
Transcranial Doppler Consultant
Menlo Park, CA 94025 USA

Camilo R. Gomez, M.D.
Associate Professor
Department of Neurology
and
Director
Comprehensive Stroke Center
University of Alabama at
  Birmingham
Birmingham, AL 35294, USA

Kathleen M. Thomas-Lukes, R.N., M.N.
Clinical Safety Specialist
Department of Safety and
  Development
Amgen, Inc.
Thousand Oaks, CA 91320-1789,
  USA

formerly:
Neuroscience Clinical Nurse
Specialist
Associate Director
Cerebral Blood Laboratory
University of California School of
  Medicine
10833 Le Conte Avenue
Los Angeles, CA 90024 USA

Library of Congress Cataloging-in-Publication Data

McCartney, John P.
    Handbook of transcranial doppler / John P. McCartney, Kathleen M.
  Thomas-Lukes, Camilio R. Gomez.
      p. cm.
    Includes bibliographical references and index.
    ISBN 0-387-94693-4 (soft: alk. paper)
    1. Transcranial Doppler ultrasonography.   2. Cerebrovascular
  disease—Ultrasonic imaging.   I. Thomas-Lukes. Kathleen M.
  II. Gomez, Camilo R.   III. Title.
      [DNLM: 1. Ultrasonography, Doppler, Transcranial—methods.
    2. Cerebrovascular Circulation—physiology.   3. Cerebrovascular
  Disorders—ultrasonography.   WL 355 M4775h 1996]
  RC388.5.M368   1996
  616.8'047543—DC20
  DNLM/DLC   96-13737

Printed on acid-free paper.

Production coordinated by Chernow Editorial Services, Inc., and managed by Natalie
Johnson; manufacturing supervised by Jacqui Ashri.
Typeset by Best-set Typesetter Ltd., Hong Kong.
Printed and bound by Edwards Brothers, Inc., Ann Arbor, MI.
Printed in the United States of America.

9 8 7 6 5 4 3 2 1

ISBN 0-387-94693-4   Springer-Verlag New York Berlin Heidelberg   SPIN 10491465

Preface

Transcranial Doppler (TCD) ultrasound, first introduced more than a decade ago, has steadily evolved into a dynamic, reliable, reproducible, and practical diagnostic tool. Clinical neuroscientists have found TCD to be an indispensable technique in the management of many types of patients. This book is designed to provide basic instruction in the performance and interpretation of transcranial Doppler ultrasonography for technologists, nurses, and physicians.

The information included in the text is critical for the development of a strong knowledge base. It is not intended to be all inclusive, and the TCD novice is likely to use it as the platform upon which to build his/her experience in the application of TCD.

This book is organized as a step-guided approach for the performance of TCD, and it includes specific guidelines for interpretation of the TCD save forms. We hope that the reader finds it useful during what we think is the most difficult phase of this technique—the learning curve.

John P. McCartney, R.V.T.
Kathleen M. Thomas-Lukes, R.N., M.N.
Camilo R. Gomez, M.D.

Acknowledgment

The authors would like to thank the following TCD manufacturers for their contributions: DWL, Medasonics, and EME/Nicolet for their contribution of the anatomy art work.

Contents

Handbook of
Transcranial Doppler

1

Introduction to Transcranial Doppler

Basic Concepts

Transcranial Doppler (TCD) ultrasound is a diagnostic technique based upon the use of a range-gated pulse-Doppler ultrasonic beam of 2 MHz frequency to assess the hemodynamic characteristics of the major cerebral arteries. The ultrasonic beam crosses the intact adult skull at points known as "windows," bounces off the erythrocytes flowing within the basal cerebral arteries, and allows the determination of blood flow velocity, direction of flow, collateral patterns, and state of cerebral vasoreactivity. Before TCD was introduced in 1982, the assessment of the cerebral arteries could only be accomplished using invasive angiographic techniques. In addition to the inherent risk that angiography carries, the information it provides is somewhat inflexible, and certainly inadequate for the moment-to-moment study of cerebral circulatory dynamics. Conversely, by sampling multiple cerebral blood vessels using TCD, it is possible to identify patterns pointing to lesions localized intra- or extracranially, follow up their natural history over time, and even monitor the effects of therapeutic strategies. Although certainly having its own inherent limitations, TCD provides physiologic information about the brain circulation that cannot be obtained by any other means. In addition to the uniqueness of the information gathered by TCD, other attractive characteristics are that it is noninvasive (i.e., safe), reproducible, versatile, and dynamic.

As noted above, the performance of TCD studies takes advantage of the existence of ultrasonic "windows." These represent specific points of the skull where the bone is sufficiently thin to allow penetration of the ultrasonic beam. Alternatively, a window may also be represented by a natural skull foramen, which serves a similar purpose. In general, performing a TCD study involves studying all possible brain vessels by insonating them through the most important ultrasonic windows, which will be further discussed elsewhere in this book.

Once the ultrasound beam has crossed the skull, it is reflected by the erythrocytes of all blood vessels in its path. Using a range-gated Doppler ultrasonic beam, it is possible to selectively sample from vascular points located at specified distances (i.e., depths) from the ultrasound transducer. Based upon a series of criteria that will be discussed elsewhere, the sonographer can unequivocally identify the vessel from which each Doppler waveform originates. In general, each cerebral artery will be identifiable based upon the ultrasonic window being utilized, the direction in which the transducer points, the depth of the sample volume, and the direction of flow. By combining the Doppler findings obtained by having sampled all possible brain arteries, clinicians are able to arrive at specific diagnoses and use the information in the management of patients.

The Cerebral Stethoscope

The utilization of TCD in clinical practice over the last decade has made us change somewhat our concept of the role that it plays. The technique, rather than an ancillary procedure, is best conceived as a specialized "stethoscope" that allows clinicians to "listen" to the hemodynamic changes of the brain blood vessels, and to compare the findings over time. Indeed, the best approach to TCD is to consider it an extension of the clinical examination, analogous to the way in which electromyography has been regarded for many years. From the clinical point of view, TCD is an ideal tool not only for diagnosis, but also for follow-up. Just as cardiologists have previously performed sequential auscultatory examinations of patients, looking for new murmurs that would alert to the development of valvular dysfunction, it is also possible to use TCD to alert us about the presence of hemodynamic disturbances representative of cerebrovascular pathology.

Applications of TCD

The clinical context in which TCD was introduced was the detection of vasospasm in victims of aneurysmal subarachnoid hemorrhage. Since then, however, there has been an explosion in its utilization in a variety of clinical and research scenarios. Time and time again the versatility of TCD has prevailed, and the technique has been able to show aspects of various clinical disorders, which previously were not fully understood. In 1990, the American Academy of Neurology issued a position paper in which the accepted applications of TCD were listed. At that time, these applications included:

1. Detecting severe (>65%) stenosis of the basal cerebral arteries.
2. Assessing the patterns of collateral circulation in patients with known severe stenosis or occlusion.
3. Evaluating and following patients with vasoconstriction of any cause, particularly following subarachnoid hemorrhage.
4. Detecting arteriovenous malformations and studying their major supply arteries and flow patterns.
5. Assessing intracranial velocity and flow changes in patients with suspected brain death.

At the time of this book's writing, a second panel of experts has been convened by the AAN to update that position statement. The following paragraphs encompass a brief review of some of the most common, current, and important applications of TCD.

Intracranial Atherosclerosis

Atherosclerosis of the cerebral vasculature is by no means restricted to the common carotid bifurcation. In fact, the second most common location of atherosclerotic plaques in the carotid circulation is the cavernous portion of the internal carotid artery. Intracranial atherosclerotic stenosis is relatively common in blacks and Orientals, and can certainly alter the prognosis and management of patients in whom it is discovered. Until TCD became available, intracranial stenoses could only be documented and followed by cerebral angiography. This is not the case any more, because TCD provides a noninvasive way of screening and following these patients.

Characteristically, TCD shows that the intracranial stenotic vessel displays increased blood flow velocities to levels greater than two standard deviations of normal. In addition to local stenosis causing increased velocities in the vessel affected, other patterns of collateralization may be identified. The intracranial vessel most easily and widely studied is the middle cerebral artery, in which stenosis and even occlusion patterns have been described. In some instances, recanalization of the occluded vessel has also be documented. The typical finding in middle cerebral artery occlusion is failure to obtain its signal, together with increased velocities in the ipsilateral anterior and posterior cerebral arteries. In some cases, however, if the occlusion is sufficiently distal, a drumbeat signal can be obtained by TCD proximal to the point of occlusion.

The Effect of Extracranial Atheromata

Lesions causing significant hemodynamic narrowing of the extracranial portions of the cerebral blood vessels cause decreased blood flow velocities. The degree of the decrement depends upon the existence of collateral flow through the communicating arteries. Such a pattern, in turn, will be characterized by increased blood flow velocities in the vessel acting as the collateral supplier. Additionally, it is possible to show reduced vasoreactivity in the hemisphere ipsilateral to the stenosis. In cases of critical carotid artery stenosis, or occlusion, typical patterns may include reversed ipsilateral anterior cerebral artery flow, increased contralateral anterior cerebral artery flow, and reversed ipsilateral ophthalmic artery flow (with internalization of the waveform).

Cerebral Vasospasm

The diagnosis of vasospasm by TCD depends upon the finding of velocities greater than two standard deviations of normal, in the appropriate clinical context. Vasospasm, in any circumstance, is a very dynamic process that requires multiple serial evaluations for its documentation and follow-up. It is because of these characteristics that TCD is so useful in the assessment of patients with vasospasm. The test should be performed as soon as a condition known to be associated with vasospasm is diagnosed. This is followed by repeat TCD studies with a frequency that depends upon the condition of the patient being studied. In patients with aneurysmal subarachnoid hemorrhage or closed head injury, daily TCD studies are performed in order to identify trends that will alert the clinicians that vasospasm is developing, and that therapeutic measures should be instituted. Along these lines; TCD can also be utilized to follow up the response to treatment, particularly the institution of interventional procedures.

Arteriovenous Malformations

Although the diagnosis of arteriovenous malformations is most commonly performed by imaging procedures, TCD may assist in the assessment of the flow characteristics of anomalies greater than 2 cm in diameter. This hemodynamic evaluation may also be of importance in the assessment of the effects of certain therapeutic procedures such as embolization. Finally, TCD can also help determine the degree of dysregulation existing in the brain region where the anomaly is located, an important variable in planning its removal and preventing the hyperemic syndrome that at times follows surgical intervention.

Cerebral Circulatory Arrest

Increased intracranial pressure results in augmented resistance to flow in the cerebral arteries. This can be readily identified by TCD as the Doppler waveforms acquire a highly pulsatile contour. In this sense, TCD indirectly provides a qualitative assessment of the intracranial pressure. The maximal expression of intracranial hypertension is the cessation of cerebral blood flow, which accompanies brain death. TCD evaluation of brain dead patients yields an unequivocal Doppler waveform displaying a "reverberating" pattern. This pattern simply results from the absence of net flow per unit of time, that is, cerebral circulatory arrest.

Detection of Emboli

The capability of TCD to detect embolic particles as they traverse the cerebral blood vessels has become a subject of intense investigation, and one with a potentially significant impact upon the care of patients with ischemic brain events. Due to the differences in impedance between the embolic material and the red blood cells, the ultrasound beam is reflected with greater intensity by the former, leading to characteristic signature signals within the Doppler waveform. These signals are known as high-intensity transients (HITs) and they vary in intensity, duration, and appearance within the cardiac cycle. Not only has it been possible to detect HITs during surgical procedures that place patients at risk for cerebral embolism (e.g., carotid endarterectomy and cardiopulmonary bypass), but also at the bedside. The latter has allowed the detection of spontaneous asymptomatic emboli in patients with atrial fibrillation and

Table 1.1 Examples of different applications of TCD monitoring.

Intraoperative	Intraprocedural	Bedside
Carotid endarterectomy	Head-up tilt table	Atrial fibrillation
Open heart surgery	Cardiopulmonary resuscitation	Arterial dissection
Radical neck dissection	Electrophysiologic testing	Paradoxical brain
	Endovascular procedures	embolism

mechanical heart valves. Such a finding has carried with it the implication that cerebral embolism may occur continuously under certain circumstances, and that the factors motivating the development of symptoms have yet to be determined. Further work is being done in order to define the role of TCD in the identification of sources of embolism when multiple possible origins exist. Additionally, the technique can be combined with the intravenous injection of agitated saline solution, allowing clinicians to diagnose patent foramina ovale (PFOs) and right-to-left shunts. This opens new possibilities for the rapid assessment and diagnosis of paradoxical cerebral embolism.

TCD Monitoring

The portability and ease-of-use of TCD, together with its versatility, have made it an ideal cerebral hemodynamic monitoring tool. Its utilization in this capacity began in the operating room, particularly during carotid endarterectomy and open heart surgery. At first, TCD showed that it was possible to determine when cerebral hemodynamic compromise was occurring during surgical procedures. Lately, the capacity for detection of cerebral emboli has given TCD an even more important role in the assessment of patients at risk for cerebral ischemic compromise as the result of intraoperative embolism. From the operating room, TCD made the logical leap to bedside monitoring. At present, its use in neurologic intensive care units and stroke units is a subject of considerable interest. The different scenarios in which TCD monitoring either has been or may in the future be of assistance to the clinicians are listed in Table 1.1. As noted, some of these still require further study. However, the versatility of TCD as a monitoring tool continues to be its most important characteristic.

Selected Readings

1. Brass LM, Durerte DL, Mohr JP. Anterior cerebral artery velocity changes in disease of the middle cerebral artery stem. *Stroke*. 1989;20:1737–1740.
2. Caplan LR, Brass L, DeWitt D, et al. Transcranial Doppler ultrasound: present status. *Neurology*. 1990;40(4):696–700.
3. Petty GW, Mohr JP, Pedley TA, et al. The role of transcranial Doppler in confirming brain death: sensitivity, specificity, and suggestions for performance and interpretation. *Neurology*. 1990;40:300–303.
4. Russell D, Brucher RR, Clark WM, et al. The intensity of Doppler signal caused by cerebral emboli materials. *Stroke*. 1992;23:474.

2

Cerebral Vascular Anatomy

There are two pairs of arteries that supply blood flow to the brain, the two internal carotid and the two vertebral arteries (Fig. 2.1). All four enter the skull, penetrate the dura, and form an arterial network at the base of the brain, the circle of Willis, from which the first-order cerebral arteries arise (Figs. 2.2, 2.3).

The Carotid Circulation (Fig. 2.4)

The internal carotid artery (ICA) enters the base of the skull and traverses the carotid canal of the petrous temporal bone. The petrous portion of the ICA then travels medially and exits the bony canal, only to enter the cavernous sinus. It bends forward along the sphenoid sinus and then turns backward forming the S-shaped curve that has become known as the carotid siphon. The more proximal portion of the ICA siphon is the parasellar segment. This is followed by the genu, and then by the supraclinoid segment, where the artery penetrates the dura.

The first branch of the supraclinoid segment of the ICA is the ophthalmic artery (OA), followed by the posterior communicating artery (PCoA), and the anterior choroidal artery. The ICA then branches into the anterior cerebral artery (ACA) and the middle cerebral artery (MCA). The internal carotid artery carries the majority of blood supply to the cerebral hemisphere and to the eye.

Ophthalmic Artery

The OA is the first intracranial branch of the ICA, and it runs forward into the orbit through the optic canal. The branches of the OA connect with branches of the external carotid artery to form important periorbital anastomoses for collateral flow.

Posterior Communicating Artery

The PCoA originates from the ICA and joins the posterior cerebral artery. Blood flow through the PCoA may be in either direction, depend-

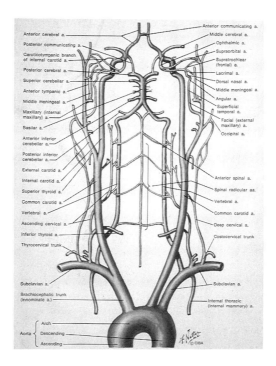

Figure 2.1 Carotid and vertebral arteries providing cerebral blood flow. Copyright © 1974. CIBA-GEIGY Corporation. Reprinted with permission from Clinical Symposia, Vol. 26, No. 1, illustrated by Frank H. Netter, M.D. All rights reserved.

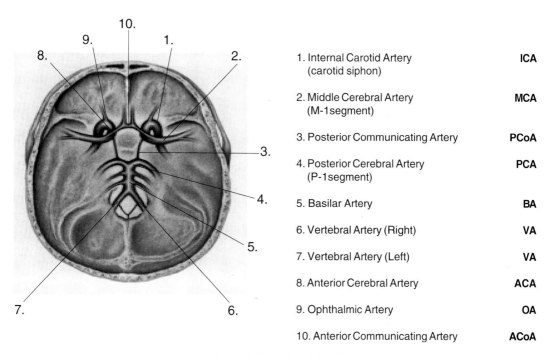

1. Internal Carotid Artery (carotid siphon)	**ICA**
2. Middle Cerebral Artery (M-1 segment)	**MCA**
3. Posterior Communicating Artery	**PCoA**
4. Posterior Cerebral Artery (P-1 segment)	**PCA**
5. Basilar Artery	**BA**
6. Vertebral Artery (Right)	**VA**
7. Vertebral Artery (Left)	**VA**
8. Anterior Cerebral Artery	**ACA**
9. Ophthalmic Artery	**OA**
10. Anterior Communicating Artery	**ACoA**

Figure 2.2 Circle of Willis.

1. Ophthalmic Artery — **OA**

2. Anterior Cerebral Artery — **ACA**

3. Middle Cerebral Artery (M-1segment) — **MCA**

4. Posterior Communicating Artery — **PCoA**

5. Posterior Cerebral Artery — **PCA**

6. Vertebro-Basilar System

7. Atlas Loop (Vertebral Artery)

8. Internal Carotid Artery (extracranial) — **EICA**

9. Carotid Siphon (intracranial internal carotid artery)

Figure 2.3 Circle of Willis: lateral view.

ing upon whether the blood supply is provided via the carotid or the vertebrobasilar systems. The PCoA is the most anatomically variable, of all the arteries in the circle of Willis, and it is often hypoplastic.

Anterior Cerebral Artery

The ACA is divided into several segments. The most proximal is known as A1 and corresponds to the portion of the ACA between its origin and its junction with the anterior communicating artery (ACoA). Distally, several segments can be identified as A2 through A5. The A1 segment of

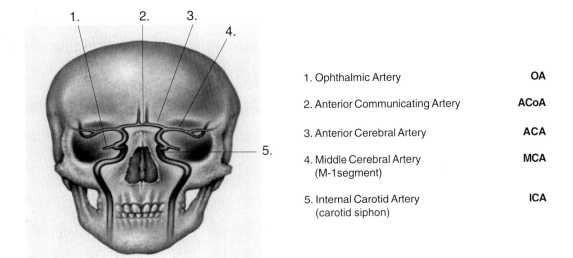

1. Ophthalmic Artery — **OA**

2. Anterior Communicating Artery — **ACoA**

3. Anterior Cerebral Artery — **ACA**

4. Middle Cerebral Artery (M-1segment) — **MCA**

5. Internal Carotid Artery (carotid siphon) — **ICA**

Figure 2.4 Carotid Arteries and anterior circulation: anterior-posterior view.

the ACA may be hypoplastic or absent. The recurrent artery of Heubner branches off the proximal A2 segment and cannot normally be assessed by TCD. The ACoA is the potential collateral source to connect both hemispheres, and is commonly hypoplastic. The distal branches of the ACA run superiorly and are not accessible to TCD examination.

Middle Cerebral Artery

The MCA courses laterally from the ICA bifurcation. It has many small collateral branches, the lenticulostriate arteries. The most proximal segment of the MCA, referred to as M1, divides into two or, less commonly, three main branches (referred to as the M2 divisions). These course superiorly and posteriorly over the convexity of the cerebral hemisphere, giving rise to distal branches. The entire M1 segment, and often part of the M2 divisions, can be studied using TCD.

The Vertebrobasilar Circulation (Fig. 2.5)

The vertebral artery (VA) is the first branch of the subclavian artery. It courses through the vertebral canal of the cervical spine prior to its entrance into the skull. The intracranial segment begins once the artery angles outward, forming a loop behind the atlas and entering the skull through the foramen magnum, piercing the dura mater. The largest branch of the VAs is the posterior inferior cerebellar artery (PICA), just proximal to the vertebral confluence. The left VA is commonly larger than the right VA, and the asymmetry can be translated into side-to-side differences in blood flow velocities. Tortuosity of the VAs may present some difficulty in the traceability of these vessels with TCD.

The basilar artery (BA) begins at the confluence of the VAs and courses anteriorly and superiorly until its bifurcation into the posterior

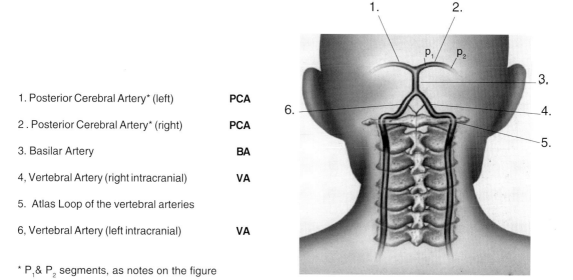

1. Posterior Cerebral Artery* (left)	**PCA**
2 . Posterior Cerebral Artery* (right)	**PCA**
3. Basilar Artery	**BA**
4, Vertebral Artery (right intracranial)	**VA**
5. Atlas Loop of the vertebral arteries	
6, Vertebral Artery (left intracranial)	**VA**

* P_1 & P_2 segments, as notes on the figure

Figure 2.5 Vertebrobasilar system and posterior circulation: posterior view.

cerebral arteries (PCA). The BA has several important branches, including the anterior inferior cerebellar artery (AICA) and the superior cerebellar artery (SCA). Insonating these branches may be misinterpreted as retrograde flow in the BA. Tortuosity of the BA is common in the elderly and requires manipulation of the transducer for maintaining proper angle of insonation.

The PCA originates from the terminal BA. The proximal segment of the PCA, from its origin to its joining the PCoA, is referred to as the P1 segment, and it courses in a plane that allows insonation through the transtemporal window. The distal P2 segment courses beyond the PCoA in a posterior and superior direction, which creates some difficulty with insonation.

Anomalies of the Circle of Willis (Fig. 2.6)

A completely intact circle of Willis is reported in only about 20% of individuals. Therefore, anomalies are more the rule than the exception. The most common anomalies are found in the ACoA, PCoA, ACA, and PCA. These vessels may be found to be hypoplastic, aplastic, or atretic.

The ACoA may be hypoplastic to the extent of impeding collateral flow. The ACA may also be hypoplastic or absent altogether. In this case, the contralateral ACA (A1) may provide blood flow to both A2 segments via the ACoA. The PCA normally originates from the BA, receiving blood flow from the vertebrobasilar system. However, the PCoA connecting the ICA to the PCA may persist as a larger vessel than the P1 segment connected to the BA. This anomaly is termed "fetal PCA" and receives blood predominantly from the ICA. The PCAs and PCoAs may be hypoplastic and limiting the collateral connection of the vertebrobasilar circulation to the carotid circulation.

The intracranial segments of the VAs may vary in length to the confluence of the BA. Consequently, this may affect the accuracy of

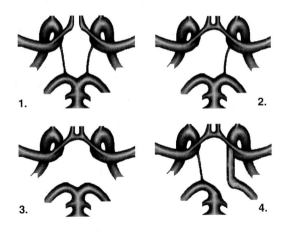

Figure 2.6 Four common congenital anomalies of the circle of Willis.

assessing the BA by measurements of the depth of insonation alone. The VAs are asymmetric in size, the left VA found to be dominant in the majority of individuals. The VAs and the BA are frequently found to be tortuous, deviating from a straight line course.

Collateral Pathways

There are several potential collateral arterial pathways, more prominent in children. In the aging population, and in the presence of hypertension, heart disease, and atherosclerosis, the number of collateral vessels decreases.

The collateral circulation in the brain is primarily established via the circle of Willis and the meningeal anastomoses. However, there are other rather complex systems that interconnect at a variety of points and that will not be covered in this text. The most common collateral connection of the two hemispheres is via the ACoA, as demonstrated angiographically (Fig. 2.7) in the presence of an occluded right common carotid artery (CCA). The right hemisphere is filled via the ACoA during a left CCA injection. Collateral flow via the ACoA may also be demonstrated with carotid compressions (Fig. 2.8). The PCoA is another potential collateral pathway, connecting the carotid and basilar vessels.

The OA is the largest and most significant communication between the external and the internal carotid arteries. In the presence of an occluded ICA, the OA can provide flow to the brain from the external carotid artery through facial–angular anastomoses. When functioning as a collateral channel, the flow direction in the OA will be reversed.

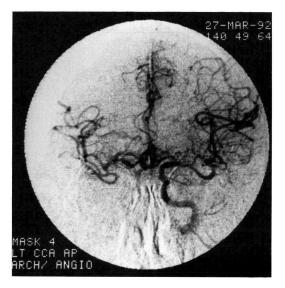

Figure 2.7 Angiogram: left common carotid injection demonstrating right hemisphere filling via the ACoA.

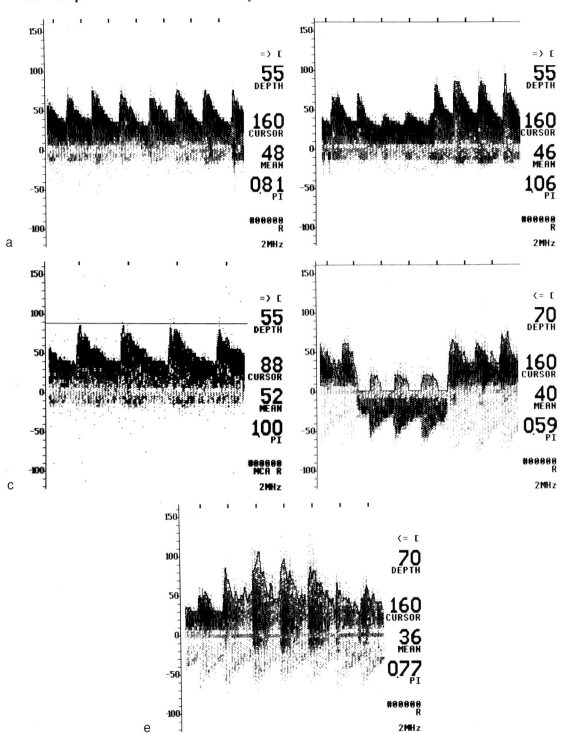

Figure 2.8 Spectral display of: (a) right MCA flow velocity; (b) diminished flow velocity right MCA during right common carotid compression; (c) slightly augmented flow velocity right MCA with left common carotid compression; (d) reversal of flow direction in right ACA with right common carotid compression; (e) augmented flow velocity right ACA with left common carotid compression.

Selected Readings

1. Baptista AG. Studies on the arteries of the brain. II. The anterior cerebral artery: some anatomic features and their clinical implications. *Neurology.* 1963;13:825–835.
2. Hutchinson EC, Yates PO. The cervical portion of the vertebral artery: a clinicopathological study. *Brain.* 1956;79:319–331.
3. Lehrer HZ. Relative calibre of the cervical internal carotid artery: normal variation with the circle of Willis. *Brain.* 1968;91:339–348.
4. Newton TH, Ptts DG (eds). *Radiology of the skull and brain, angiography; volume II, book 2: arteries.* St. Louis: C.V. Mosby; 1974.
5. Williams PL, Warwick R, Dyson M, Bannister LH (eds). *Grays anatomy.* 37th ed. New York: Churchill Livingston; 1989.

3

Doppler Basics

The utilization of TCD in clinical practice requires some fundamental knowledge about Doppler. With this in mind, the intent of this section is to introduce, in plain terms, the many technical variables and concepts encountered in TCD.

Doppler Principle

The Doppler principle, first described in 1842 by the Austrian physicist, Christian Andreas Doppler, can be defined as a change in apparent frequency due to the relative motion between the observer and the sound source. An example occurring in everyday life is the familiar change in pitch, or frequency, of a passing ambulance with siren blaring, or a passing train, with horn blowing. As the ambulance approaches, the siren grows louder and increases in pitch, but as it moves away the pitch decreases rapidly along with the intensity.

In medicine, Doppler ultrasound instruments (Dopplers) have long been used to evaluate blood flow in the peripheral vascular system. These instruments utilize transducers constructed with piezo-electric crystals that, when stimulated electrically, transmit an ultrasonic wave, and that translate ultrasound into electronic pulses. Currently operating with frequencies anywhere between 1 and 20 MHz, Dopplers have numerous applications in clinical medicine, one of them being TCD.

Doppler Formula

Doppler instruments analyze blood flow by having the sound source and the observer at same location (i.e., transducer). The Doppler ultrasound beam is transmitted and bounced off of the erythrocytes; the difference between the transmitted signal and the received signal is the Doppler shift. This is directly proportional to the velocity of the moving blood cells, and for medical purposes, the formula that illustrates it is expressed as:

$$F = \frac{2FtV\cos\theta}{C}$$

where F is the Doppler frequency shift, V is the object velocity, C is the speed of sound in tissue, and $\cos\theta$ is the correction factor.

In general, although the desired information is velocity, the equation is solved for Doppler frequency shift (in kilohertz). The reason is that Doppler instruments, without imaging guidance, do not provide the angle of incidence between the ultrasound beam and the vessel. Without knowing this angle, the correction factor cannot be determined. Consequently, the equation cannot be accurately solved for velocity.

TCD and the Doppler Formula

The same Doppler principle is used when examining blood flow velocities within the basal cerebral arteries using TCD. Here, however, a $0°$ angle of incidence (θ) is assumed between the vessel and the ultrasound beam. As such, replacing all of the constants with their relative values results in velocity being the only unsolved variable in the equation, thus reducing the equation to $F = V$:

$$F = \frac{2(2\,\mathrm{MHz})V1}{1540}$$

where $Ft = 2\,\mathrm{MHz}$, V is the velocity of blood flow, $C = 1540\,\mathrm{m/s}$, and $\cos\theta = 1$.

But why does the angle of incidence (θ) used by the equation have a magnitude of $0°$? The truth is that the magnitude of the angle is unknown, but it is assumed to be very small due to the reasons noted below.

The Effect of Angle of Ultrasonic Incidence

In TCD it is generally assumed that the angle of incidence between the ultrasound beam and the vessel is less than $30°$ and, as such, the maximal difference between measured and real velocities will not be greater than 13%. If the angle of incidence increases beyond $30°$ the measurement error increases dramatically, so when the angle of incidence reaches $45°$, the Doppler shift reflects only 70% of the real velocity ($\cos 45° = 0.30$). At $90°$, when a vessel is perpendicular to the ultrasound beam, a Doppler shift cannot be detected, at least in the theoretical sense, because the cosine of 90 is 0. This results in the reflected frequency being the same as the transmitted frequency.

Doppler Modes: Continuous vs. Pulsed Wave

Doppler transducers, when stimulated by an electrical current, emit an ultrasound signal that passes through the soft tissues of the body until reflected by moving blood cells within the arteries and veins. The reflected signal is then received by the transducer and changed back into an electrical signal. This is referenced to (subtracted from) the transmitted signal, and amplified and processed in various ways. The two most common are audible analysis and Fast Fourier Transformation (FFT). The first allows the examiner to hear flow in a blood vessel and the second, also known as spectral analysis, allows for visual display and further analysis of the signal.

Two basic modes of Doppler technology are available in clinical medicine. Continuous wave (CW) Doppler involves the steady passage of an electrical current through the piezoelectric material of the transducer to produce one continuous wave of ultrasound. On the other hand, pulsed wave (PW) Doppler functions by having intermittent bursts, or pulses, of electrical current stimulate the piezoelectric material to produce intermittent ultrasound waves.

Although both CW and PW Dopplers operate with the same transmission frequencies, and even process the received Doppler signal in the same way, their construction differs significantly (Figs. 3.1, 3.2, 3.3). To start, CW Doppler systems operate using two piezoelectric crystals in the transducer. One crystal sends the ultrasound signal, while the second crystal receives the reflected signal. Conversely, PW Doppler systems operate with only one crystal in the transducer. This is alternately stimulated to produce the ultrasound signal, and then dampened (made quiet) to "listen" for the returning signal. The key to PW Doppler function is the creation and control of the electronic pulse that stimulates the transducer, and the opening of a receiving gate to listen for the reflected signal.

Comparing the internal workings of the two instruments reveals that a CW Doppler contains an oscillator that sends a signal to an output amplifier and a mixer, whereas the oscillator of a PW Doppler sends a

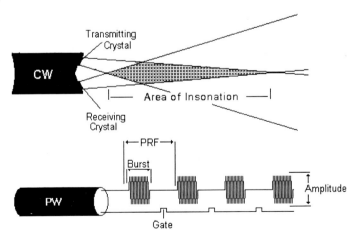

Figure 3.1 CW/PW transducer comparison.

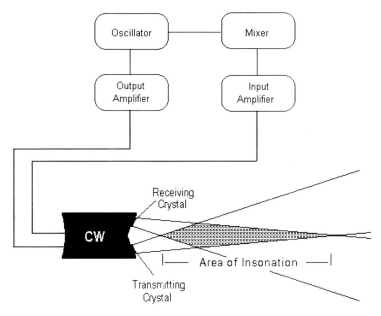

Figure 3.2 CW Doppler construction.

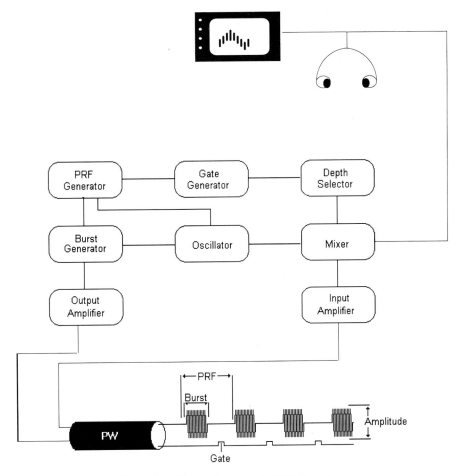

Figure 3.3 Block diagram of a PW Doppler.

signal to both a pulse repetition frequency (PRF) generator and burst generator, as well as a mixer, making it significantly more complex (Figs. 3.2, 3.3). Uses, advantages, and disadvantages of both CW and PW Dopplers are provided in Table 3.1.

When examining the peripheral vasculature, transducer selection is dependent on two things: depth of the vessel being evaluated and need to control the transmitted signal. Depth of the vessel under investigation determines the operating frequency of the transducer, whereas the need to control the transmitted signal determines the type of transducer used (CW vs. PW). In TCD, low-frequency PW transducers, usually operating in the range of 2 MHz, are used for three reasons: first, relatively deep structures need to be analyzed; second, low-frequency ultrasound is needed to penetrate the cranium; third, PW transducers have the added benefit of allowing for the control of sample volume size and depth of analysis. Without this control, analysis of the basal cerebral arteries would not be possible.

Signal Generation, Power Output, and the Doppler Signal

At the heart of every PW Doppler system lies an oscillator. Responsible for the origin of the Doppler signal, it sends an electronic pulse to three components: the burst generator, PRF generator, and a mixer. Of these, the burst generator and the PRF generator are involved with signal

Table 3.1 CW/PW comparison.

CW Doppler
   Advantages
   - **Large area of insonation, which allows for easier analysis of blood flow through vessels within the range of the Doppler's capabilities. (The examiner is not required to know the exact depth at which to analyze an artery or vein, as long as it lies within the depth of the Dopplers capabilities.)**
   - **Aliasing is not a problem as there is no pulse repetition frequency to contend with.**

   Limitations
   - **Only sensitive where transmitting beam and reflected beam overlap, which creates a dead area between the transducer surface and the area of insonation where signals cannot be analyzed.**
   - **No control of depth.**
   - **No control of sample volume.**
   - **Spectral display contains information from any movement strong enough to create a Doppler shift in the area of insonation. As such, the signal may reflect multiple vessels.**

PW Doppler
   Advantages
   - **Defined sample volume size allows for discrete analysis of a vessel segment.**
   - **Depth control allows for the analysis of signals from shallower or deeper depths as necessary.**

   Limitations
   - **Aliasing.**
   - **The higher the scale setting, the shallower the depth of penetration.**

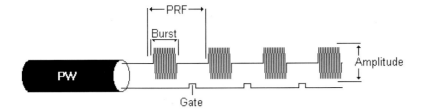

Figure 3.4 PW Doppler demonstrating ultrasonic pulse transmission. The operator adjusts controls as necessary to do an examination. At the same time those controls "adjust" the transducer operation and power output.

generation and contribute to ultrasound power output, whereas the mixer references the incoming signal to the transmitted signal in order to realize the extent of the Doppler shift. Processing of the Doppler shifted signal is discussed below. In this section, the role of each component contributing to signal generation is discussed. Not only will we address the Doppler signal created, but also the adjustment and control of ultrasound power output (Fig. 3.4). This is done because of the ALARA (as low as reasonably allowable) guideline recommended by the Food and Drug Administration (FDA).

PRF Generation and Scale Adjustment

The TCD examiner thinks in terms of scale adjustment, but this is controlled by the PRF generator. When the scale is adjusted to accommodate higher velocities, the PRF generator increases the number of pulses transmitted over a given period of time (Fig. 3.5). As such, increasing the scale automatically increases the ultrasound power output, unless this is compensated in some other way (e.g., lowering the signal amplitude). If, on the other hand, the scale is lowered, the ultrasound power output decreases as the PRF decreases. To maintain a strong signal when the scale is lowered, either the amplitude of the transmitted signal or the gain of the incoming signal must be increased. In terms of the ALARA principle, it is better to boost the power output only when necessary and, if possible, to compensate for weaker signals first by increasing gain. In addition, an inverse relationship can be seen between depth and the ability to analyze maximum velocities. Consequently, at greater depths of analysis, only lower scale settings will be available for use. The reason

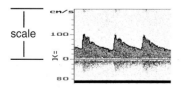
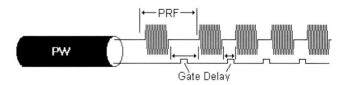

Figure 3.5 Increasing "scale" increases the number of pulse transmissions over a given period of time, thereby increasing power output. Correspondingly, the time between pulse transmissions shortens, resulting in less time to wait for signals returning from deeper vessels.

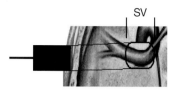
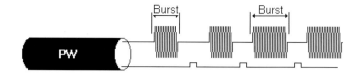

Figure 3.6 Adjusting sample volume (SV) determines the length of the pulse transmission, which in turn increases or decreases power output. The larger the sample volume, the longer the burst and the greater the power output.

is that, in order to analyze signals from greater depths, the time delay before opening the receiver gate must be significantly increased.

Burst Generation and Sample Volume Adjustment

The size of the sample volume, measured along the axis of the ultrasound beam, is controlled by the burst generator. In general, larger sample volumes result from longer pulse transmission (measured in microseconds) and, thus, result in greater power output (Fig. 3.6).

Output Amplifier and Signal Intensity

The output amplifier controls the strength of the transmitted signal, or signal intensity (Fig. 3.7). It does not affect either the PRF or the burst length in any way, but it is usually used to compensate for changes in either of these two. In view of this, if the power output displayed on a particular TCD system does not change when the scale or sample volume is changed, then it is most likely that an automatic intensity adjustment is built into the system to compensate for this. Although this makes things easier for the operator, it also removes some of the operator's control. Following the ALARA principle, unless a strong signal is needed to penetrate thick craniums, it is best to reduce the signal intensity when increasing the scale or increasing the sample volume.

Gain Control

Unlike adjustments in scale, sample volume, or signal intensity, gain does not affect ultrasound power output. This is because gain adjustment only affects the strength of the incoming signal. Consequently, when more powerful signals are transmitted, less gain is required to process the

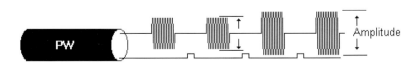

Figure 3.7 Adjusting "amplitude" increases or decreases the strength of the pulse transmission, which in turn increases or decreases the power output.

received signal. Gain should always be adjusted according to the image on the FFT display, as discussed below. Following the ALARA principle, when a stronger signal is required, gain is the ideal first adjustment. However, if the incoming signal remains weak, then the power output of the transmitted signal must be increased as the system allows.

Gate Generator and Depth Adjustment

After the pulse is transmitted, the system must wait for the signal to travel to the desired depth and back, which is expressed as:

$$t = 2\,d/c$$

where t is the time to wait, d is the desired depth, and c is the speed of sound in tissue (approximately 1540 m/s).

Depth is measured from the transducer to the center of the sample volume and is adjusted using an electronic receiving gate, which opens to accept the reflected signals. The delay in opening this gate corresponds to the signal returning from the desired depth. Figure 3.8 demonstrates that deeper analysis requires a longer delay in opening the receiving gate whereas analysis of shallower depths requires a shorter gate delay.

A new technique, multirange gating, allows for the simultaneous analysis of signals from multiple depths. This is accomplished by opening a series of gates as demonstrated in Figure 3.8b.

Signal Processing

FFT analysis, or spectral analysis, provides a way of presenting three-dimensional Doppler data in a two-dimensional format. With spectral

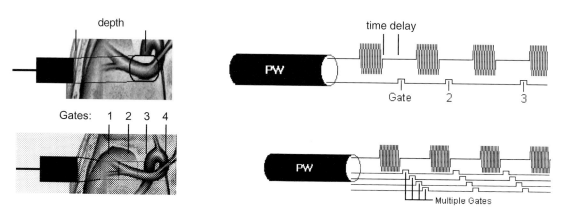

Figure 3.8 (a) Range gating (adjusting depth) is accomplished by "adjusting" the time delay between transmitting the ultrasound burst and opening the gate to receive signals. Analyzing signals from shallower depths requires a short relay(2), where long delays (3) are necessary to analyze signals from deeper vessels. (b) Multiple-range gating is accomplished by opening a series of receiving gates to enable the system to "receive" information from multiple depths simultaneously. In this example, information is analyzed from four depths simultaneously by opening a series of four receiving gates.

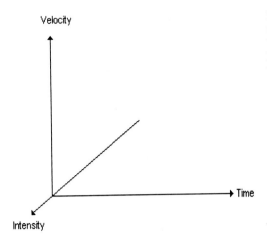

Figure 3.9 Spectral analysis (FFT analysis) results in three dimensions of data displayed in two dimensions. Velocity is displayed on the vertical scale, time on the horizontal scale, and signal intensity (amplitude) as the brightness of a point.

analysis time is displayed on the horizontal scale, velocity (or frequency) on the vertical scale, and signal intensity is displayed as relative brightness (Fig. 3.9). But before examining how the FFT data are displayed, it is helpful to understand the makeup of the matrix onto which they are projected.

FFT Display Matrix

Magnifying an FFT display, as in Figure 3.10, reveals that it is composed of a row of columns of points with each FFT column representing one discrete moment in time while the number of FFT columns in the display is determined by the length of the display. The number of points per FFT

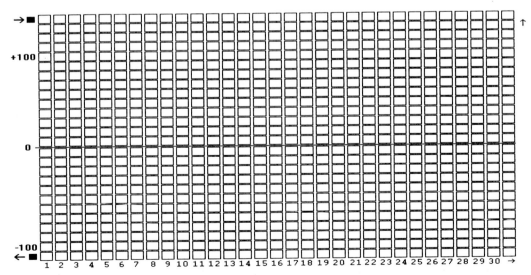

Figure 3.10 Matrix of a 26-point FFT display, demonstrating flow toward the transducer above the zero line and flow away from the transducer below the zero line. Each column of points represents one moment in time (1 FFT). Thus, time is displayed on the horizontal scale and velocity on the vertical scale. Signal intensity (brightness of each point) has not yet been registered.

Figure 3.11 FFT resolution: The greater the number of FFT points the greater the spectral resolution.

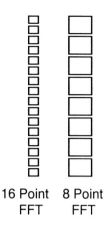

16 Point   8 Point
FFT   FFT

column, measured from the bottom to the top of the column, is dependent on the FFT resolution: the higher the value, the better the resolution. Figure 3.11 compares the spectral resolution of 8 and 16 points of FFT. In TCD, spectral displays range from 64 to 256 points of FFT.

Also, in order to demonstrate flow toward and away from the transducer, a zero line is placed on the horizontal axis near the center of the display. Finally, a velocity scale is added. In addition, many TCD systems also have either a color or gray scale indicating the signal decibel resolution as explained below.

FFT Data

The received Doppler information is contained in a signal composed of various amplitudes measured using the decibel scale as depicted in Figure 3.12. The signal displayed in the figure represents one moment in

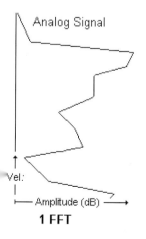

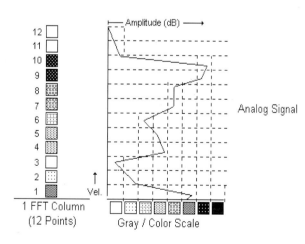

Figure 3.12 (a) Analog display of the Doppler signal for one column of FFT. Velocity is displayed on the vertical scale and signal amplitude, measured using the decibel scale, is displayed on the horizontal scale. (b) In this example, the Doppler signal is then analyzed using a matrix composed of a 12-point FFT column and a color or gray scale composed of 8 shades. The color assigned to each point of the FFT column corresponds to the signal strength, measured in dB as determined by the gray color scale.

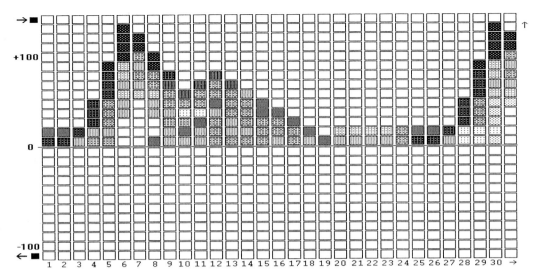

Figure 3.13 Matrix of the same 26-point FFT display (Fig. 3.10), now registering signal intensity as brightness of each point in the FFT column.

time and is analyzed in this example, using a matrix composed of 12 points of FFT on the vertical scale (velocity) and eight shades of color or gray on the horizontal scale (signal amplitude). A color/gray scale value is assigned to each point in the FFT column according to the strength of the signal at that velocity. Thus, when viewing the FFT column (Fig. 3.12) and comparing it against the color/gray decibel scale it can be seen that the strongest signals were recorded at points 9 and 10 whereas the weakest signals were recorded at points 11 and 12. All other points in the FFT column lay somewhere in between. As the Doppler instrument gathers information, this same analysis is made for each FFT column in the display. Upon completion of the spectral display sweep, regularities corresponding to velocity changes through out the cardiac cycle should appear (Fig. 3.13). If the received signal were displayed in the decibel analysis format (Fig. 3.14), a velocity profile would still be seen, but the compilation of it would be more difficult to ascertain and minute changes

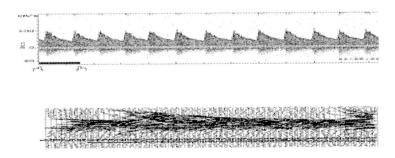

Figure 3.14 Top: example of a full spectral display sweep. Bottom: analog display of the Doppler signal for the first cardiac cycle. Velocity is displayed on the vertical scale and signal amplitude, measured using the decibel scale, is displayed on the horizontal scale in addition to time.

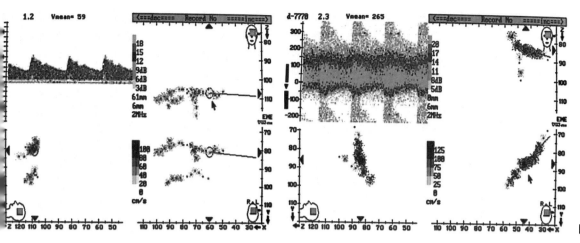

Figure 3.15 (a) Example of spectra from a normal vessel. (b) Example of a spectra from a stenosis with lower intensity signals registering at the high-est velocities and higher intensity signals at lower velocities throughout the rest of the cardiac cycle.

more difficult to interpret. Consequently, an FFT display is both easier to view and easier to understand.

When interpreting patient data it is important to remember that, for signals not containing emboli, the color/gray scale value assigned to a particular point in the FFT column reflects the signal amplitude, itself a reflection of the percentage of blood flowing at that velocity in the sample volume. For example, a signal from a normal vessel may appear with randomized colors throughout the FFT column below the envelope curve (Fig. 3.15a), whereas the signal from a high-grade stenosis or vasospasm may display low-intensity signals at the highest velocities and high-intensity signals at the lowest velocities (Fig. 3.15b). In general, the FFT display is capable of revealing:

- uniform blood flow (velocity profiles appearing uniform with good cross-representation of color or gray),
- turbulence (high-intensity, low-velocity signals),
- artifact or air embolus* (uniform spike of high-intensity color from bottom to top of spectral display),
- particulate embolus (high-intensity signals within the spectral display).

Embolus Detection and FFT Data

Perhaps the newest field of research in TCD is that of embolus detection. Essentially, the application of TCD here is based upon the theory that the Doppler signal reflected from a particle (fat, blood clot, etc.) travel-ing through the blood stream should be significantly stronger than that from normal blood flow. The term high-intensity transient signals

---

*Spectral displays with inadequate decibel resolution register both artifact and air embolism as the same. This is due to signal overload.

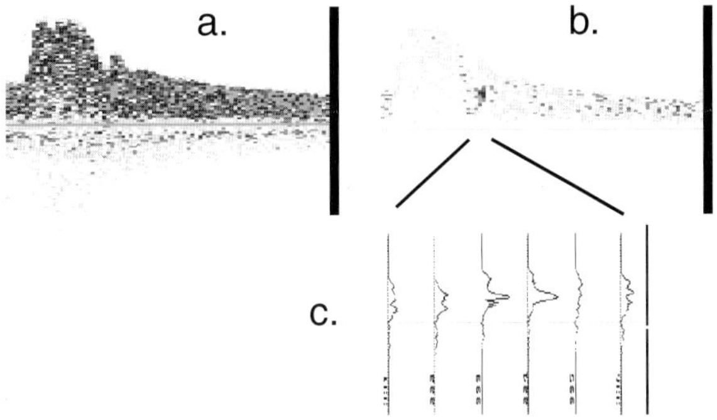

Figure 3.16 (a) FFT display of TCD signal with normal gain setting showing one cardiac cycle. (b) Same spectra with gain reduced, revealing the embolus. (c) Display of the analog, dB, presentation of the embolus. Note the higher decibel spikes in the two FFT columns where the embolus occurs.

(HITS) was coined along the way as an identifier of the Doppler footnote of potential embolic material. When setting system parameters for embolus detection it is important to set the signal threshold (trigger) at a level that blocks out as much artifact as possible while allowing the stronger, potential embolus, signals through. Figure 3.16a,b demonstrates the effect of gain adjustment on the FFT display of a cardiac cycle containing an embolus, while Figure 3.16c shows the corresponding amplitude spike of the signal.

Display Resolution and Embolus detection

Considering that an embolus signature may involve relatively few points of FFT and extend as few as one or two FFT columns, it is important to address areas of FFT display resolution that may be overlooked in routine TCD examinations: FFT, time, and decibel resolution.

If, for example, TCD is used to evaluate vasospasm and the question is to use either a 64- or 128-point FFT display, a 64-point FFT display, practically speaking, provides the same mean velocity data as 128- or even 256-point FFT. In embolus detection, however, higher FFT resolution may have a decided advantage. Decibel resolution determines the quality of the spectral image of the FFT display. FFT displays with lower decibel resolution are overloaded earlier than FFT displays with higher decibel resolution. Time resolution is determined by the speed of the Doppler board, number of points of FFT, and other hardware and software. Basically, the faster the system the better the time resolution, while allowing for greater FFT resolution.

Maximum Velocity Follower (Envelope Curve)

The envelope curve (maximum frequency follower) is a line drawn electronically on the FFT display corresponding to the maximum velocity of the cardiac cycle in each FFT column. Upon completion of the FFT sweep, in order to obtain accurate data (mean velocity, PI, etc.), this line should follow, as close as possible, the maximum velocities of every cardiac cycle for the entire sweep. In other words, it should "envelop" each cardiac cycle.

Some systems derive the envelope curve by measuring from the top of the spectral display down to the first strong incoming signal, others measure from the zero line out to the last strong incoming signal, and still others use a different technique for deriving the envelope curve all together. Regardless of the method used, it is important to have proper gain adjustment, particularly if derivation of the envelope curve is tied to intensity (strength) of the displayed signal. Figure 3.17 demonstrates that too much gain may result in the maximum frequency follower analyzing noise whereas too little gain, with a poor signal, may result in velocities analyzed well below the envelope of the cardiac cycle.

In routine TCD evaluations, where the goal is the measurement of mean velocity, after the envelope curve is derived the FFT data is virtually ignored, as it is from the envelope curve that mean velocity, pulsatility index (PI), and even systolic and diastolic velocities are measured. The spectral display, however, still provides important information about potential spectral broadening, turbulence, and emboli.

Diagnostic Parameters

Two types of mean velocity can be discussed in regards to TCD. One is an intensity-weighted mean velocity, which is derived by averaging the different amplitudes of the FFT column, while the other is a time-averaged, area-averaged, mean velocity value derived by placing a line on the horizontal axis of the envelope curve of the cardiac cycle so that the area above the line V_1 is equal to the area below the line V_2 (Fig. 3.18). Of the two, the time-averaged mean velocity is certainly more universally accepted, and is the mean velocity used in this guide.

Of the most widely known derivations of PI, the most commonly accepted is Gosling's formula (Fig. 3.19):

$$ PI = \frac{V_{max} - V_{min}}{V_{mean}} $$

where V_{max} is the peak systolic velocity, V_{min} is the end diastolic velocity, and V_{mean} is the mean velocity.

Aliasing

The speed at which ultrasound pulses are transmitted (and received) determines the highest Doppler frequency shift, or velocity, that can be detected. Remembering that the speed at which the pulses are transmitted is called the PRF, the Nyquist principle tells us that the highest Doppler frequency shift that can correctly be determined is one half the PRF. Any received velocities (frequencies) greater than that produces aliasing.

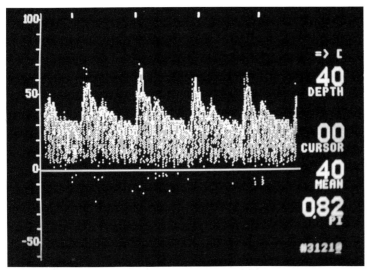

a

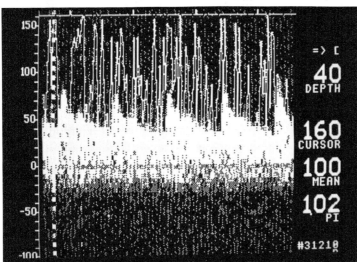

b

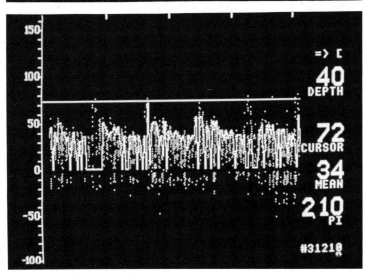

c

Figure 3.17 (a) FFT display with optimal gain setting, envelope curve follows outline of cardiac cycles. (b) FFT display with gain too high, envelope curve spikes to noise. (c) FFT display with suboptimal gain, envelope curve drops to zero line.

Figure 3.18 Mean velocity is calculated by placing a line along the horizontal axis of the envelope curve (maximum frequency follower), so that the areas of V_1 equal the areas of V_2. The value produced is both time-averaged and area-averaged. Some refer to this as the mean of the maximum velocities.

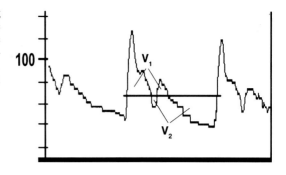

Figure 3.19 Pulsatility index (Gosling) is calculated by subtracting the end diastolic velocity from the systolic velocity, and dividing the remainder by the mean velocity. The value produced is a ratio of peak systolic velocity to end diastolic velocity and is currently important when evaluating signals from patients with increased intracranial pressure. It is important to note, however, that many other factors, such as CO_2 concentrations in the blood, also affect PI.

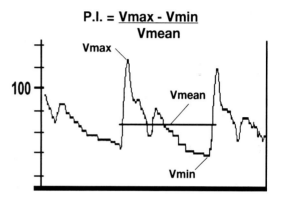

The concept of aliasing can be explained using an analogy. If the blade of a fan, marked with a piece of tape, turns at 60 rpm, or once a second, and a camera shutter records the movement, then according to the Nyquist principle, the camera shutter must open faster than 0.5 s to record the movement accurately. If a camera shutter is set to open every 0.33 s while the fan, described above, turns in a clockwise rotation at 60 rpm, the rotation will be recorded accurately. That is, the rotation appears clockwise with the event recorded accurately every 0.33 s (Fig. 3.20). Now, if the camera shutter speed is slowed to every 0.5 s, every time the shutter opens the marked fan blade appears to be in one of two positions: top dead center or bottom dead center. As such, a bistable display is produced. The result is that direction cannot be determined (Fig. 3.21). If the camera shutter is set to open even slower (e.g., every 0.66 s), the movement will be incorrectly recorded in a reverse direction (Fig. 3.22).

In TCD, if the Doppler shifted frequency is more than one half the RPF then the FFT data reaching the limit of the display is cut off and folded over, appearing incorrectly as high-flow velocities spiking in the opposite direction (Fig. 3.23a). To compensate, the examiner may increase the PRF by increasing the scale (Fig. 3.23b), or, if unable to do so because of the depth/PRF limitation. The zero line can be lowered. This electronically cuts the aliasing information from the bottom of the FFT display and electronically pastes it at the top of the display (Fig. 3.23c).

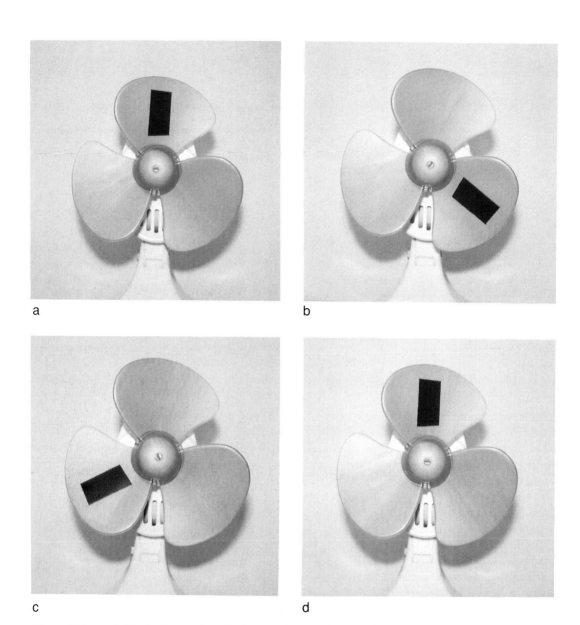

Figure 3.20 (a–d) Clockwise rotation of a fan noted correctly using shutter speeds of 0.33 s while fan turns at 60 rpm.

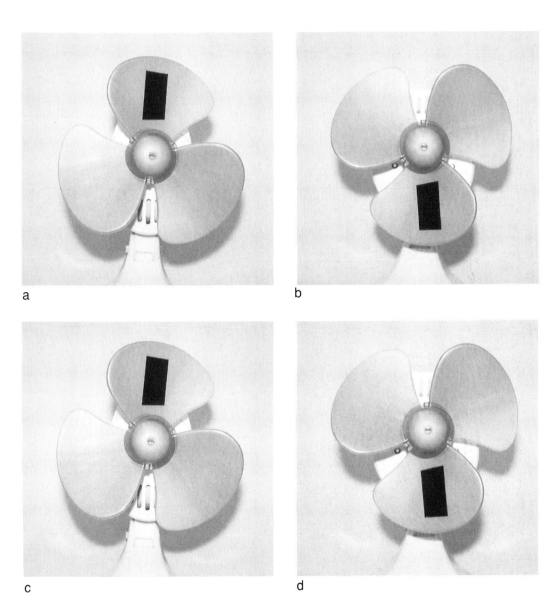

Figure 3.21 (a–d) Clockwise rotation of a fan recorded incorrectly because the shutter speed of 0.5 s while fan turns at 60 rpm is too slow; as a result aliasing occurs.

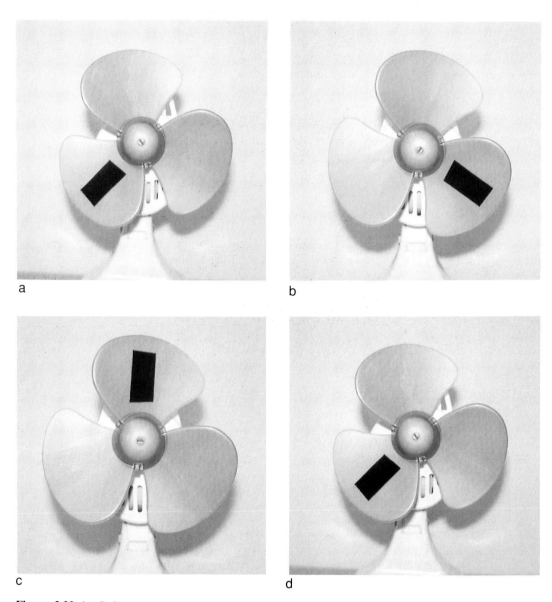

a

b

c

d

Figure 3.22 (a–d) Incorrect counterclockwise rotation of a fan noted because the shutter speed of 0.66 s, while fan turns at 60 rpm is too slow; as a result aliasing occurs.

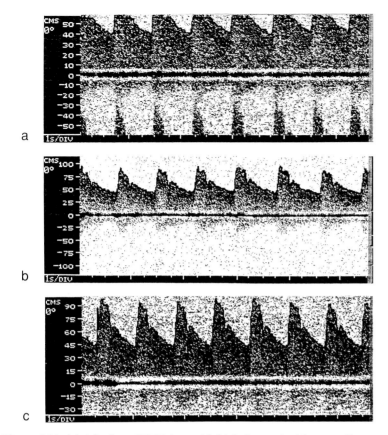

Figure 3.23 (a) Aliasing of FFT data with high-flow velocities cut off at top and spiking up from the bottom of the display. (b) Aliasing solved by increasing scale. (c) Aliasing compensated for by lowering the zero line.

Selected Readings

1. Aaslid R. The Doppler principle applied to measurement of blood flow velocity in cerebral arteries, in *Transcranial Doppler sonography*. Wien: Springer-Verlag; 1986:22–38.
2. Barnes RW. Continuous wave Doppler ultrasound, in *Noninvasive diagnostic techniques in vascular disease*. St. Louis: C.V. Mosby Co.; 1985:19–24.
3. Beach KW, Strandness DE Jr. Pulsed Doppler ultrasound for blood velocity measurements, in *Noninvasive diagnostic techniques in vascular disease*. St. Louis: C.V. Mosby Co.; 1985:20–32.
4. Berger MP, Tegeler CH. Embolus detection using ultrasonography, in *Transcranial Doppler sonography*, Babikian, VL, Wechsler LR (eds). St. Louis: C.V. Mosby; 1993:232–241.
5. Bode H. Introduction to Doppler sonography, in *Pediatric applications of transcranial doppler sonography*. New York: Springer-Verlag; 1988:11–15.
6. Burns PN. *Doppler ultrasound: principles, current status and future potential*. Ottawa: CSVT; 1992.
7. Carstensen EL. Acoustic cavitation and the safety of ultrasound. *Ultrasound Med Biol*. 1987;13(10):597–606.
8. Eden A. *The search for Doppler*. New York: Springer-Verlag; 1992.

9. Evans DH, McDicken WN, Skidmore R, Woodcock JP. *Doppler ultrasound: physics, instrumentation, and clinical applications.* London: John Wiley & Sons Ltd.; 1989.

10. Kremkau FW. *Diagnostic ultrasound, principles, instrumentation, and exercises,* 2nd ed. New York: Grune & Stratton Inc.; 1984:5–31, 123–138.

11. Kremkau FW. Ultrasound principles review: Doppler artifacts II. *J. Vasc. Technol.* 1990;14(3):123–124.

12. Moehring M. *Introduction to physics and instrumentation of Doppler ultrasound; basic tutorial.* Cerebral Hemodynamics Annual Meeting; 1994.

13. Reid JM. *Cerebrovascular evaluation with Doppler ultrasound.* The Hague: Martinus Nijhoff Publishers bv; 1981:23–40, 41–48, 57–68.

14. Russell D. The detection of cerebral emboli using Doppler ultrasound: theoretical, experimental, and clinical aspects, in *Transcranial Doppler*; Newell DW, Aaslid R (eds). New York: Raven Press; 1992:207–213.

15. Spencer M. *Detection of cerebral arterial emboli; transcranial Doppler,* Newell DW, Aaslid R (eds). New York: Raven Press; 1992:215–230.

16. Strandness DE Jr. Doppler ultrasonic techniques in vascular disease; *Noninvasive diagnostic techniques in vascular disease.* St. Louis: C.V. Mosby Co.; 1985:13–18.

4

Essential Cerebrovascular Hemodynamics

The introduction of transcranial Doppler (TCD) has allowed for a relatively basic understanding of cerebral hemodynamics. The technique has made evident the important effect of many variables, such as resistance, intracranial pressure (ICP), variations in partial pressure of carbon dioxide (CO_2), and cerebral perfusion pressure (CPP), on cerebral blood flow velocities. The following is an overview of the most fundamental hemodynamic principles of TCD.

Ohm's Law

Ohm's law, originally derived from the physical principles of electrical circuits, has also been applied to vascular hemodynamics in order to describe the relationship between pressure, resistance, and flow. In this context, Ohms law is translated as flow = pressure/resistance.

Generally, if resistance remains constant and pressure increases, flow increases. If, however, pressure remains constant and resistance increases, flow decreases. The application of Ohm's law to cerebrovascular hemodynamics is reflected in the formula: cerebral blood flow = cerebral perfusion pressure/cerebrovascular resistance.

If cerebral perfusion pressure (CPP) remains constant and cerebrovascular resistance (CVR) increases then cerebral blood flow (CBF) decreases. Viewed along these lines, the pressure–flow–resistance relationship is such that, any change in CVR must be matched by a proportional change in CPP in order for CBF to remain constant. Conversely, changes in CPP generally lead to proportional changes in CVR in order to regulate the CBF. This mechanism is known as autoregulation and will be discussed later.

Cerebral Perfusion Pressure

Cerebral Perfusion Pressure (CPP) is the driving force of flow within the intracranial circulation. Mathematically, it is expressed by the formula:

$$CPP = MABP - \text{ICP}$$

where *MABP* is mean arterial pressure and *ICP* is intracranial pressure.

In general, reductions in MABP or increases in ICP have a similar effect upon CPP, they lower it. This effect translates into characteristic changes in the TCD waveform: Vmean decreases and pulsatility increases (Fig. 4.1).

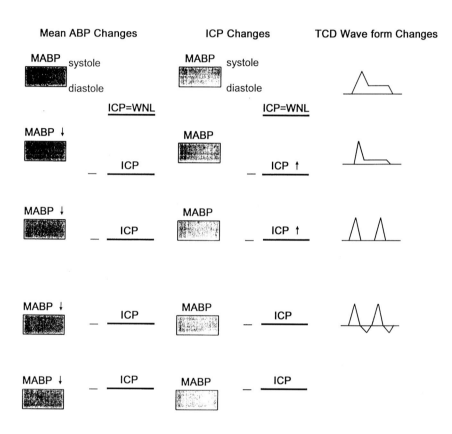

MABP = Mean Arterial Blood Pressure
ICP = Intracranial Pressure

Figure 4.1 Under normal conditions, end diastolic velocity is about one half of systolic velocity and ICP is well below mean arterial pressure. However, when ICP increases, or when MABP decreases, the first observable effect is that end diastolic velocity decreases. When ICP equals diastolic pressure, flow in diastole is absent. As ICP continues to rise, or MABP continues to fall, peak systolic velocity decreases and flow in diastole, instead of continuing to flow into the vessel, flows out of the vessel. The extent of this to-and-fro flow is directly related to ICP and MABP, and the wave form morphology can take on many different appearances. It is important to note that to-and-fro flow is not restricted to increased ICP but has been reported at the moment of aneurysm rupture. A special type of to-and-fro flow may also occur in subclavian steal given the right circumstances.

Cerebrovascular Resistance

The flow of fluids through rigid tubes is governed by Poiseuille's Law, which is expressed mathematically as:

$$Q = \frac{\Delta P \, \pi \, r^4}{L8\eta}$$

where Q is the flow, ΔP is pressure gradient, π is the 3.1412, L is the length of vessel segment, η is the viscosity of blood, and r^4 is the radius raised to the 4th power.

Using Poiseuille's formula as a basis, it is possible to derive the formula for resistance as follows:

$$R = K\left(\frac{8\eta L}{\pi r^4}\right)$$

Where R is the resistance, K is the mathematical constant equal to or greater than 1 (1 representing a minimal loss of flow with a parabolic profile), η is the viscosity of blood, L is the length of the vessel segment, π is the mathematical constant of 3.1412, and r is the radius.

In relation to flow and resistance, Poiseuille's law demonstrates three things:

- Resistance is directly proportional to the viscosity of blood (η)
- Resistance is directly proportional to the length of the vessel segment.
- Resistance of a vessel is inversely proportional to the vessel radius raised to the fourth power (diameter squared).

These statements underscore the fact that, under normal physiologic conditions, change in vessel diameter represents the most significant factor that affects resistance. The fact that the relationship between a vessel's cross-sectional area and resistance is represented by r^4 indicates the magnitude of the effect of vascular diameter changes in the control of blood flow.

Cerebral Resistance Vessels

Under normal circumstances, blood flows from arteries to arterioles, capillaries, venules and, finally, into collecting veins. As long as ICP remains normal, most of the resistance in the cerebrovascular circulation is provided by the arterioles and their precapillary sphincters (Table 4.1).

Table 4.1 Distribution of resistance throughout the vascular system.

3%	63%	21%	7%	6%
arteries	arterioles	capillaries	venules	veins

From Ref. 13.

In turn, the basal cerebral arteries that form the circle of Willis, under normal circumstances, play only a very minor role in determining cerebrovascular resistance. This is an important concept in the use of TCD, because it implies that the vessels readily accessible to evaluation have a relatively constant diameter throughout the examination. The role of arterioles (vessels with a resting diameter of 50 μm or less) in the regulation of cerebrovascular resistance stems from their ability to dilate and constrict in response to the vasomotor action of smooth muscles. The magnitude of their effect, in light of Poiseuille's Law, is enormous, and a slight constriction or dilation of their diameter has a radical effect upon CPP and, at times, on CBF.

Cerebral Autoregulation and Vasomotor Reactivity

Autoregulation is the ability of the cerebrovascular system to maintain CBF independently of changes in CPP. As with any other physiologic system, the autoregulatory mechanism has limits within which it performs. For most individuals, as long as CPP remains between 60 and 160 torr, CBF remains constant.

Cerebral autoregulation can be assessed at the bedside using TCD in conjunction with a variety of techniques. One of which involves the inflation and subsequent deflation of blood pressure cuffs, placed on the upper thighs, while continuously monitoring MCA velocities and MABP. Deflation of the thigh cuffs produces a sudden drop in MABP and, consequently, in CPP. A comparison is then made between changes in the TCD velocities and the return of the MABP to baseline. Normal autoregulation demonstrates a prompt return of MCA flow velocities, before the return of the blood pressure to baseline. However, in patients with impaired autoregulation the TCD velocities passively follow changes in MABP.

Alternately, the effects of changes in partial pressure of carbon dioxide (CO_2) upon TCD velocities can be utilized to test the reactivity of the cerebral arterioles, even though, strictly speaking, this is not equal to autoregulation. As stated earlier, the assumption is that the diameter of the MCA remains relatively constant, while the resistance vessels (vasomotor arterioles) change in caliber through vasodilatation and constriction. In general, hypercapnia results in vasodilation of the vasomotor arterioles. This, in turn, decreases the artery/arteriole pressure gradient allowing an increase of flow throughout the system (Fig. 4.2). This increase in flow is observable in the basal cerebral arteries as an increase in velocity and a decrease in P.I. when monitored with TCD (Fig. 4.2b). Conversely, hypocapnia leads to constriction of the vasomotor arterioles with increased distal resistance and ultimately a decrease in cerebral blood flow. This is reflected in a lower mean velocity and increased P.I. (Fig. 4.2c). CO_2 reactivity studies provide important information about the reserve capacity of patients in a variety of circumstances, as discussed elsewhere in this book.

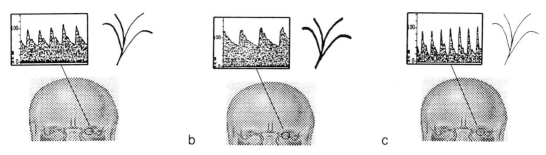

Figure 4.2 (a) MCA recording with resting (steady-state) flow velocities and PI. (b) MCA recording demonstrating the effect of vasodilatation causing increased velocities and reduced PI. (c) MCA recording demonstrating the effect of vasoconstriction causing decreased velocities and increased PI.

The Effects of Stenosis

The velocities measured by TCD directly reflect the hemodynamic changes occurring in the vessel segment being studied (i.e., point of insonation). In general, the relationship between the important variables involved is given by the formula: $Q = V \times A$. Where Q is the flow, V is the velocity, and A is the cross-sectional area. It follows that, if flow is to remain constant in the presence of a stenotic lesion, mean velocity *must* increase. Furthermore, the mathematical relationship between the variables is such, that a diameter reduction of 30% results in doubling the baseline mean velocity. In turn, a diameter reduction of 50% leads to a quadrupling of the mean velocities. Understanding this mathmatical relationship is important, even though it does not take into account the dynamic aspects of cerebrovascular reactivity (see above). Further, it is only applicable to instances of single, focal lesions, and is only valid under conditions in which flow remains constant despite the stenosis (i.e., to a maximum of 60–70% diameter stenosis).

Poiseuille's law (Fig. 4.3) assumes the existence of laminar flow. However, as luminal diameter decreases, laminar flow becomes turbulent and

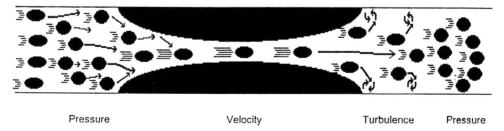

Pressure   Velocity   Turbulence   Pressure

Figure 4.3 The Bernoulli effect explains that an increase in velocity in a stenosis is inversely proportional to the reduction in area of the lumen of the vessel. Flow across the stenosis, however, results in a change of energy from potential energy, proximally, to kinetic energy across the stenosis and back to potential energy distally. In a theoretical sense this energy conversion does not result in an energy loss. The Bernoulli effect does not, however, take into account the turbulence that occurs when flow exits a stenotic lesion.

Bernoulli formula: $\Delta P = 1/2\rho(V_2^2 - V_1^2)$, where ΔP is the pressure gradient, ρ is the density of blood, V_2 is the velocity in the stenosis, and V_1 is the initial velocity.

is characterized by the presence of swirls and eddies. In such circumstances, flow is approximately proportional to the square root of the pressure gradient rather than to the pressure itself. Downstream turbulence offers additional local resistance.

Selected Readings

1. Aaslid R, Lindegard K-F. Cerebral hemodynamics, in *Transcranial Doppler Sonography*, Aaslid R (ed). Wien: Springer-Verlag; 1986:60–85.
2. Carter SA. Hemodynamic considerations in peripheral and cerebrovascular disease, in *Introduction to vascular ultrasonography*, Zwiebel WJ (ed). Orlando, FL: Grune & Stratton, Inc.; 1982:23–40.
3. Giller CA, Bowman G, Dyer H, Mootz L. *Diameter changes in cerebral arteries during craniotomy*. 5th International Symposium on Intracranial Hemodynamics, Feb 1991; San Francisco, CA.
4. Gosling RG, King DH. Continuous wave ultrasound as an alternative and complement to X-rays in vascular examination, in *Cardiovascular applications of ultrasound*, Reneman RS (ed). Amsterdam: North-Holland; 1978:266–282.
5. Grote E, Hassler W. The critical first minutes after subarachnoid hemorrhage. *Neurosurgery*. 1988;22:654–661.
6. Hassler W, Steinmetz H, Gawlowski J. Transcranial Doppler ultrasonography in raised intracranial pressure and in circulatory arrest. *J. Neurol.* 1988;68:745–751.
7. Müller HR, Casty M, Moll R, Zehnder R. Response of middle cerebral artery volume flow to orthostasis. *Cerebrovas. Dis.* 1991;1:82–89.
8. Newell DW, Grady M, Sirotta P, Winn HR. Evaluation of brain death using transcranial Doppler. *Neurosurgery*. 1989;24:509–513.
9. Planiol T, Pourcelot L. Doppler effect study of the carotid circulation, in *Ultrasonics in Medicine*, de Vlieger M, White DN, McCready VR (eds). New York: Elsevier; 1973:104–111.
10. Ringelstein EB, Sievers C, Ecker S, Schneider PA, Otis SM. Noninvasive assessment of CO_2-induced cerebral vasomotor response in normal individuals and patients with internal carotid occlusions. *Stroke*. 1988;19:963–969.
11. Ringelstein EB. A practical guide to transcranial doppler sonography, in *Noninvasive imaging of cerebrovascular disease*. New York: Alan R. Liss, Inc.; 1989:75–121.
12. Spencer MP, Arts T. Some hemodynamical aspects of large arteries, in *Doppler ultrasound in the diagnosis of cerebrovascular disease*, Reneman RS, Hoeks APG (eds). Chichester, England: John Wiley & Sons Ltd.; 1982:59–75.
13. Zijlstra WG. Physiology of the cerebral circulation, in *Cerebral blood flow, basic knowledge and clinical implications*, Minderhoud JM (ed). Amsterdam: Excerpta Medica; 1981:34–55.
14. Ringlestein EB, Otis S. Physiologic Testing of Vasomotor Reserve, In *Transcranial Doppler*, Newell DW, Aaslid R, (eds). New York: Raven Press, 1992, pp. 83–97.

5

Examination Techniques

Cranial Windows

There are three natural occurring ultrasonic "windows" in the cranium. They comprise locations where the bone is sufficiently thin to allow penetration with the ultrasound beam, or are located where natural foramina serve the same purpose. Each cranial window allows blood flow velocity to be measured from a different group of arteries. Using the sound of the Doppler signal as a feedback, the ultrasonographer can mentally construct an image of the intracranial arteries, and their position in relation to the incident beam. While insonating each vessel, adjustments in the transducer position and angle allow sampling from different points along the arterial system. The ultrasonic cranial "windows" which are used for insonation of the major intracranial arteries are the transtemporal, transforaminal or suboccipital, and transorbital windows. In addition, a fourth approach, retromandibular, should also be used for a complete assessment.

Transtemporal (Fig. 5.1)

This window allows direct assessment of the middle cerebral artery (MCA), the anterior cerebral artery (ACA), the posterior cerebral artery (PCA), and the terminal segment of the internal carotid artery (TICA). In addition, when the posterior (PCoA) and anterior communicating arteries (ACoA) function as collateral channels it is also possible to reach conclusions about their patency.

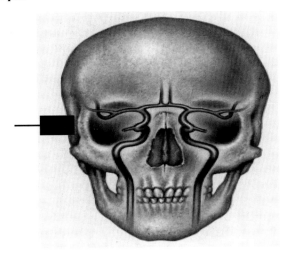

Figure 5.1 Transtemporal approach, used for evaluating the MCA, ACA, PCA, and TICA, including ACoA, and PCoA, if providing collateral flow.

Transforaminal or Suboccipital (Fig. 5.2)

This window allows assessment of the suboccipital (V3) and intracranial portions (V4) of both vertebral arteries (VA) and of the basilar artery (BA).

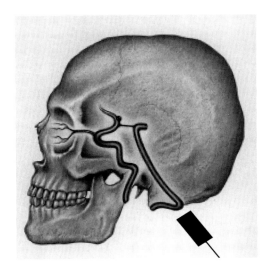

Figure 5.2 Foraminal (suboccipital) approach, used for evaluating the vertebral and basilar arteries.

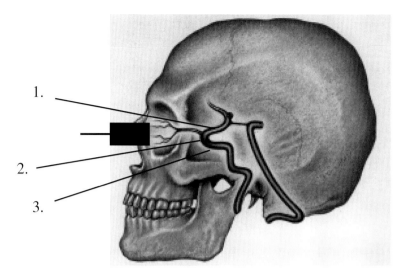

1.

2.

3.

Figure 5.3 Transorbital approach, used for evaluating the ophthalmic artery and carotid siphon (1, supraclinoid; 2, genu; 3, paracellar).

Transorbital (Fig. 5.3)

This window allows assessment of the ophthalmic artery (OA) and the internal carotid artery siphon (ICA) (i.e., cavernous segment of the ICA).

Retromandibular (Fig. 5.4)

Technically this is not a cranial window but an extracranial approach for assessing the distal segment of the extracranial ICA, just before it enters the skull base. The velocity measurement obtained in this segment of the ICA is important in distinguishing vasospasm from hyperemia, in moni-

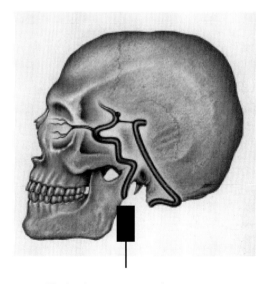

Figure 5.4 Retromandibular (submandibular) approach, allows for evaluation of the distal extracranial ICA.

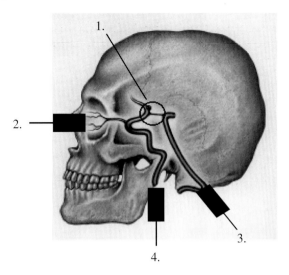

Figure 5.5 The three approaches used in evaluating the circle of Willis, plus retromandibular approach (1) Transtemporal approach: evaluation of MCA, ACA, PCA, TICA, ACoA, and PCoA, if providing collateral flow. (2) Transorbital approach: evaluation of ophthalmic artery and carotid siphon. (3) Foraminal (suboccipital) approach: evaluating the vertebral and basilar arteries. (4) Retromandibular approach: evaluation of distal portion of the extracranial ICA.

toring changes in flow volume in patients with arteriovenous malformations (AVM), and in the detection of ICA dissection.

When performing a complete transcranial examination, all of these windows must be utilized to provide a comprehensive assessment of the cerebral arteries (Fig. 5.5).

The TCD Study

The TCD probe is range-gated, allowing for insonation of the cerebral arteries at several selected depths. Velocity measurements may therefore be recorded at various points throughout the entire arterial segment, increasing the likelihood of detecting focal pathologic processes. Both velocity and flow direction are recorded and used for identification of each artery. Pulsatility or resistance indices are also recorded and are helpful for interpreting flow patterns. Velocities from the basal cerebral arteries in normal subjects have been reported by various authors. (Table 5.1). In general, the normal values are greatly reproducible between different laboratories.

The performance of TCD studies relies completely on the understanding of the cerebrovascular anatomy, physiology, hemodynamics, and the experience of the ultrasonographer. A mental image of the intracranial arteries may be constructed by a skilled ultrasonographer as the study is performed.

Ideally, the patient should be resting in a supine position; the TCD instrument may be placed on either side of the patient. The ultrasonographer may choose to be seated behind the patient's head, or stand in a manner that allows comfort and support of the hand holding the transducer. Stereo headphones provide the best method for critically

Table 5.1 Criteria for identification of basal cerebral arteries using TCD.

Window	Vessel	Depth	Normal V_m	Direction of flow*
Transtemporal	MCA	45–55	60 ± 12	toward
	ACA	55–75	50 ± 12	away
	PCA	65–80	40 ± 11	toward/away
Transorbital	OA	30–55	20 ± 10	toward
	ICA	55–70	50 ± 15	toward/away
Transforaminal	VA	65–85	40 ± 10	away
	BA	>85	40 ± 10	away

* In relation to transducer.
MCA = middle cerebral artery; ACA = anterior cerebral artery; PCA = posterior cerebral artery; OA = ophthalmic artery; ICA = internal carotid artery; VA = vertebral artery; BA = basilar artery.

listening to the Doppler signal, particularly in noisy environments.

While first learning the technique of TCD, ultrasonographers are tempted to look at the monitor screen to watch for the spectral image, and to ignore the probe position over the cranial window. We find it more practical to maintain the eyes fixed on the position of the probe, while listening to the sounds of the Doppler signal. This method allows us to make small adjustments in the position and angle of the probe, using an audio feedback approach. Once the best quality and loudest of the audible signals is obtained, it is possible to visually verify the quality of the Doppler spectrum. Furthermore, intently watching the monitor while ignoring the probe position may cause the probe to easily slip completely off the proper window. Also, adjustment of the probe based upon listening to the changes in the audible signal allows the ultrasonographer to quickly identify the proper orientation for achieving the best signal, facilitating subsequent studies performed on the same patient.

It is extremely important to perform each examination in a systematic, standardized fashion, to assure accuracy in vessel identification. Velocity measurements should be obtained in 2 mm steps throughout each arterial segment, in order to accurately trace the vessel and to reliably identifying bifurcations and changes in flow direction.

Transtemporal Window Examination

The transtemporal window is located over the temporal bone, just superior to the zygomatic arch. This window can be located in one of three different positions: posterior, middle, and anterior (Fig. 5.6). While assessing the intracranial circulation, each of these areas should be explored for the best Doppler signal. Utilizing the anterior window requires a more posterior angulation of the probe, while utilizing the posterior window requires angling the probe more anteriorly (Fig. 5.7).

Initially, the middle area of the temporal window is investigated for an audible Doppler signal. This is the easiest, most common, and best window in young patients. It is found halfway between the outer canthus and the external auditory meatus, above the zygomatic arch. The probe is positioned flat against the skin with a slight anterior and superior orientation. The posterior temporal window is located just in front of the external auditory meatus, and above the zygomatic arch. It allows the

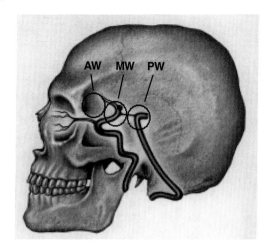

Figure 5.6 Location of transtemporal windows: AW = anterior window; MW = middle window; PW = posterior window.

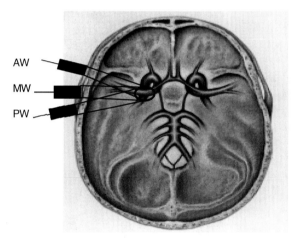

Figure 5.7 Orientation of the transducer to the MCA for the transtemporal approach: AW = anterior window; MW = middle window; PW = posterior window.

best ultrasound penetration in the older population and may be the only area in which an audible Doppler signal may be obtained. When the posterior area of the temporal window is utilized, the probe will require an anterior orientation. The anterior temporal window is found slightly higher than the previous two, and slightly closer than the middle window to the outer canthus. The probe will require a posterior orientation for insonation of the intracranial arteries (Fig. 5.7).

Middle Cerebral Artery (Fig. 5.8)

The MCA can be insonated through the transtemporal window at depths between 35 and 65 mm and it displays flow directed toward the probe. The mean blood flow velocity (MBFV) is normally 60 ± 12 cm/s, depending upon the patient's age and the physiologic factors that influence the velocity (Table 5.2). For completeness, the entire segment of the MCA should be assessed, to decrease the likelihood of overlooking focal pathology. The error introduced by the Doppler angle is one of MBFV "reduction." Therefore, the highest MBFV obtained should be recorded and used for interpretation.

Middle Cerebral Artery Characteristics:

Depth	35-65mm
Direction	Toward the transducer
Window	Temporal, Anterior/Superior

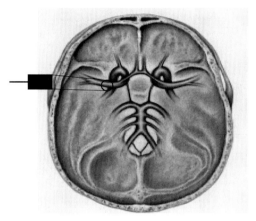

50
DEPTH   160

78
MEAN

0.87
PI⁺

> ■   0
FLOW

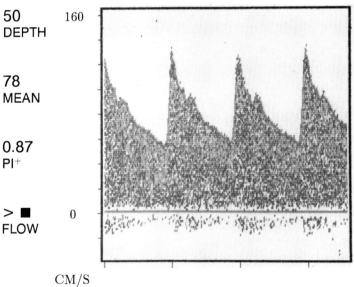

CM/S

Figure 5.8 Insonation of the MCA.

Table 5.2 Factors influencing velocity.

Physiological factor	Effect upon MBFV
Age	< with increasing age
HCT	Inverse relationship
P_{CO_2}	> with increasing P_{CO_2}
Metabolic demand	> with increased metabolism
Gender	female > male

ICA Bifurcation (Fig. 5.9)

Continuing through the transtemporal window, usually at a depth of 60 to 65 mm, there is either an abrupt change in the direction of flow or a bidirectional pattern. The bidirectional or "butterfly" waveform spectrum one sees indicates the bifurcation of the terminal ICA into its two cranial branches, the MCA (M1 segment) and the ACA (A1 segment). A slight anterior–superior orientation of the probe allows more precise assessment of the A1 segment.

MCA / ACA Bifurcation Characteristics:

Depth	60-65mm
Direction	MCA = Toward / ACA = Away
Window	Temporal, Anterior/Superior

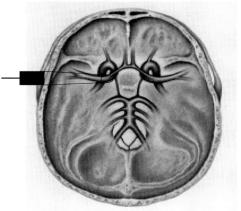

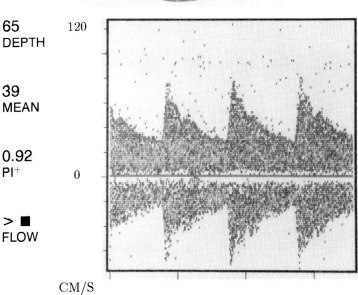

65
DEPTH

39
MEAN

0.92
PI+

> ■
FLOW

120

0

CM/S

Figure 5.9 Insonation of the MCA/ACA bifurcation.

Terminal Internal Carotid Artery (Fig. 5.10)

The velocity of the TICA can be measured at depths between 60 and 65 mm, again displaying flow directed toward the probe. The MCA and the ICA waveform spectra are difficult to separate at this depth, because only a slight change in the probe angle will move the Doppler sample volume from one artery to the other. An inferior orientation of the probe position over the temporal window is best for obtaining the most accurate velocity recording of the TICA, its normal MBFV ranging 50 ±

Terminal Internal Carotid Artery Characteristics:

Depth	60-65mm
Direction	Toward
Window	Temporal, Inferior

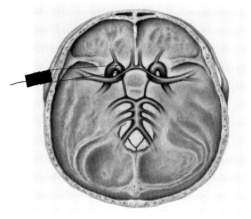

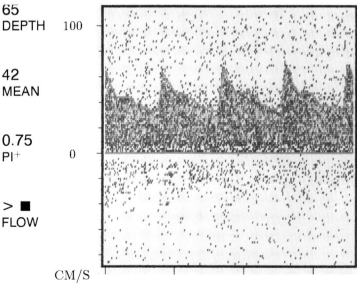

Figure 5.10 Insonation of the terminal ICA.

12 cm/s. Velocity measurements of the TICA are the least accurate, due to an anatomically poor angle of insonation.

Anterior Cerebral Artery (Fig. 5.11)

The A1 portion of the ACA can be assessed in its entirety at depths between 60 and 80 mm. The direction of flow in the ACA is normally away from the ipsilaterally placed probe. At the brain's midline, approximately at a depth of 80 mm, it is common to observe a bidirectional

Anterior Cerebral Artery Characteristics

Depth	60-75mm
Direction	Away
Window	Temporal, Anterior / Superior

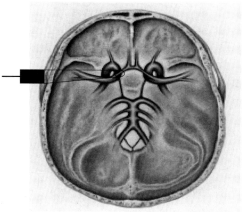

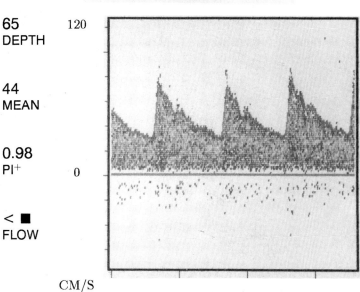

65
DEPTH

44
MEAN

0.98
PI+

< ■
FLOW

CM/S

Figure 5.11 Insonation of the ACA (A1 segment).

Doppler waveform, representative of both ACAs as they converge. This is due to the relatively large sample volume in relationship to the two vessels (Fig. 5.12). The normal MBFV in the ACA is 50 ± 12 cm/s. However, this can be significantly different if the ACA is utilized as a collateral channel, or if the vessel is hypoplastic. The A2 portion of the ACA cannot be properly assessed using TCD, generally because of its location and course.

ACA Midline Characteristics

Depth	75-80mm
Direction*	Away / Toward
Window	Temporal, Anterior / Superior

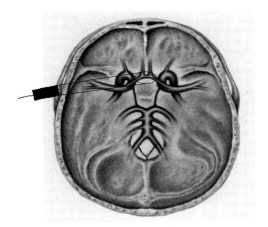

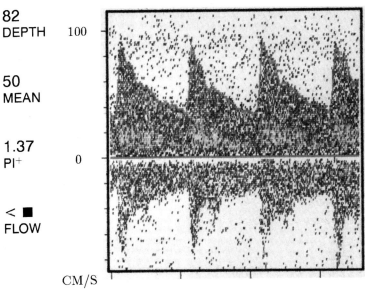

82
DEPTH   100

50
MEAN

1.37
PI+   0

< ■
FLOW

CM/S

Figure 5.12 Insonation of the ACAs at midline. *When insonating the ACA at midline, the flow signal will reflect either one or both of the ACAs. This is due to the relatively large sample volume in relation to the close proximity of the two vessels and the short ACoA.

Posterior Cerebral Artery (Fig. 5.13)

The PCA can be found by aligning the transducer slightly posteriorly and inferiorly from the point of the ICA bifurcation. Beginning at a depth of 60 to 75 mm, its P1 segment is found to show a direction of flow toward the transducer. It is often possible to also sample the P2 segment (i.e., distal to the PCoA) by changing the orientation of the transducer laterally. The flow direction in the P2 segment is normally away from the probe, and bidirectional Doppler waveforms (i.e., simultaneous sam-

Posterior Cerebral Artery Characteristics

Depth	60-75mm
Direction	Toward
Window	Temporal, Posterior / Inferior

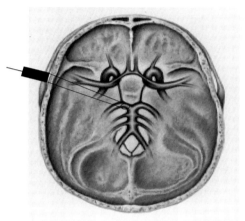

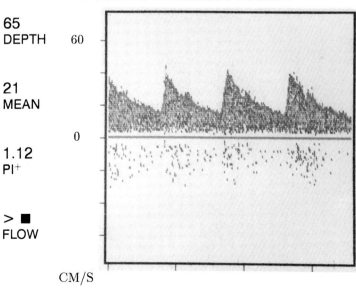

65 DEPTH	60
21 MEAN	
	0
1.12 PI⁺	
> ■ FLOW	

CM/S

Figure 5.13 Insonation of PCA (P1 segment).

pling of P1 and P2 segments) can be recorded in the curve of the PCA. In addition, following the P1 segment to the midline will lead to another bidirectional waveform reflecting both P1 origins: the bifurcation of the BA. Again, this is due to the relatively large sample volume in comparison to the PCAs (Fig. 5.14). The normal MBFV of the PCA is 40 ± 10 cm/s, regardless of which of its two segments is sampled.

PCA (Midline) Characteristics

Depth	75-85mm
Direction*	Toward / Away
Window	Temporal, Posterior / Inferior

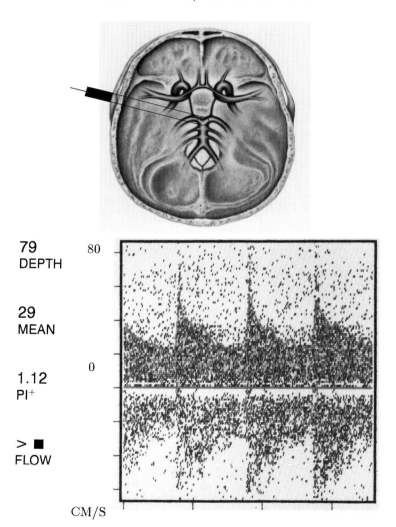

Figure 5.14 Insonation of the PCAs at midline. *When insonating the PCAs at midline, the flow signal may reflect either one or both vessels. This is due to the relatively large sample volume as well as the bifurcation of the BA into the right and left PCA.

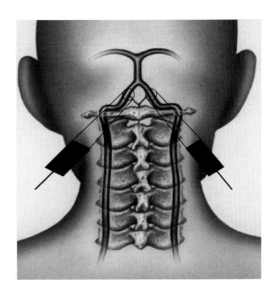

Figure 5.15 Insonation of the vertebral arteries with probe position posterior to mastoid region.

Transforaminal/Suboccipital Window

The transforaminal or suboccipital window is located at the most superior and posterior portion of the neck (Fig. 5.15). The ultrasound beam passes between the atlas (i.e., first cervical vertebra) and the base of the skull. In order to be able to insonate the vertebrobasilar circulation, the patient should be positioned on his/her side, allowing the ultrasonographer complete visualization of the neck area. If this is not possible, removal of the pillow and turning of the patient's head away from the side of investigation will allow the probe to be slipped under the neck while the patient is supine. For patients who are ambulatory and who can fully cooperate, a sitting position is often the best for complete accessibility of the neck area and recording of the velocities.

Vertebral Artery

The VAs are assessed individually by angling the probe to the right and left of the midline (Fig. 5.16). We recommend starting with the right VA, orienting the probe to the right, and at a depth of 65 mm. The Doppler waveform identified at this point may be directed toward or away from the transducer, or it may be bidirectional. The reason for this variation is that the VA exits the vertebral canal and it is first directed posteriorly, only to curve inwardly and then follows an anterior–superior course. The entire VA can be assessed to its most distal portion, at a depth of approximately 85 mm, where it joins the contralateral VA to form the BA. The normal MBFV in the VA is in the range of 40 ± 10 cm/s. Asymmetry in the vertebral velocities is not uncommon, and it is usually due to congenital asymmetry of the two vessels. The left VA is dominant in 45% of the population whereas the right is dominant in 21% of individuals.

Figure 5.16 Insonation of the left (a) and right (b) VA.

Vertebral Artery Characteristics:

Depth	65-85mm
Direction	Away
Window	Foramen Magnum / Suboccipital

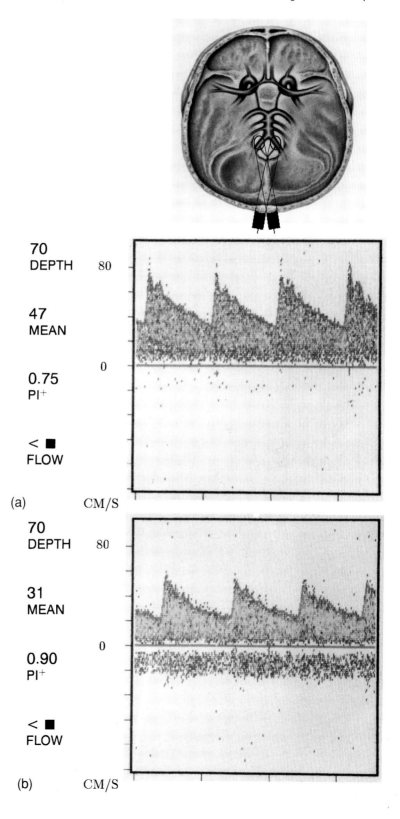

Basilar Artery

By increasing the depth of the sample volume while following the VAs to their confluence, it is possible to assess the proximal portion of the BA (Fig. 5.17). Usually, the BA can be followed from its origin, approxi-

Basilar Artery Characteristics:

Depth	85-120mm
Direction	Away
Window	Foramen Magnum / Suboccipital

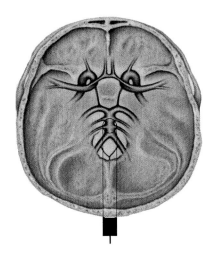

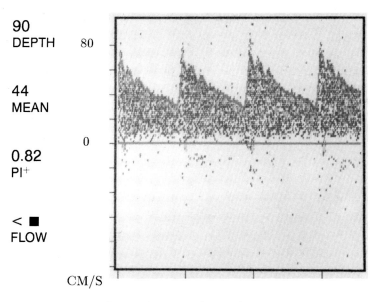

90
DEPTH   80

44
MEAN

0.82
PI+

< ■
FLOW

CM/S

Figure 5.17 Insonation of the BA.

mately 85 mm deep, up to a depth of 120 mm. While tracing the BA distally, the signal may become attenuated due to ultrasound absorption, and the probe may need to be placed more inferior on the neck and pointed more superiorly to maintain the best Doppler signal. Imagine the probe to be a flash light that is angled in such a way as to shine the beam of light through the foramen magnum to the patient's nose. The MBFV normally recorded in the BA should be within 40 ± 10 cm/s, with the flow directed away from the transducer.

Transorbital Window

In order to take advantage of this window, the transducer is placed directly over the closed eyelid. The patient should be instructed to gently close his/her eyes, but to avoid squinting. A small amount of gel should be applied directly over the closed eyelid. Contact lenses do not need to be removed. However, hard contact lenses may cause discomfort when slight pressure with the transducer is applied over the eyeball. This part of the exam should not be done if the patient has recently had surgery for implantation of an intraocular lens, as the effects of ultrasound on a newly implanted lens are unknown. The power of the TCD instrument should be decreased to approximately 20% of its maximum during insonation through the transorbital window.

Ophthalmic Artery (Fig. 5.18)

The ophthalmic artery is the first supraclinoid branch of the ICA, and runs extracranially into the orbit. The importance of assessing the ophthalmic artery relates to its collateral functions, as this artery connects with the branches of the external carotid artery. Under normal circumstances, flow through the OA is directed toward the transducer. When the ICA is either occluded or critically narrowed, flow reversal in the OA will underscore its function as a collateral channel. The depth at which the OA can be identified varies between 45 and 60 mm. The direction of flow is normally toward the transducer and velocity normally approximates 20 ± 10 cm/s. The Doppler waveform of the OA shows high pulsatility because this vessel supplies blood flow to a muscular arterial bed of high resistance.

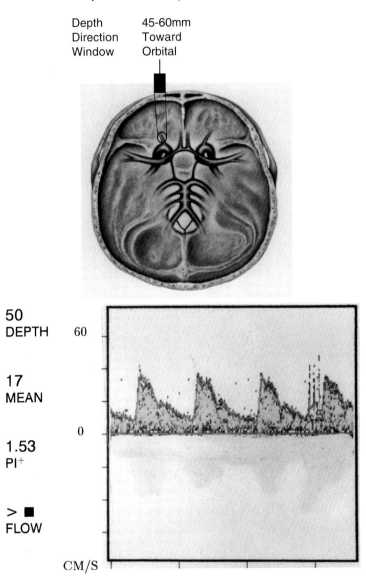

Ophthalmic Artery Characteristics:

Depth   45-60mm
Direction   Toward
Window   Orbital

50
DEPTH   60

17
MEAN

1.53
PI⁺

> ■
FLOW

CM/S

Figure 5.18 Insonation of the OA.

ICA Carotid Siphon (Fig. 5.19)

The carotid siphon can also be assessed through the transorbital window by increasing the depth of the sample volume. The direction of flow varies among its various segments, being toward the probe Fig. 5.19 in the parasellar portion (below the genu), bidirectional in the genu, and away from the probe in the supraclinoid portion. The Doppler waveform of the ICA siphon is quite different from that of the OA, being more consistent with a low-resistance cerebral artery. The ICA siphon is initially assessed at a depth of 60 mm, and can be traced as deep as 75 mm. The normal velocity in the ICA siphon is approximately 50 ± 12 cm/s.

Carotid Siphon Characteristics:

Depth	60-75mm
Direction	Toward / Away (bidirectional)
Window	Orbital

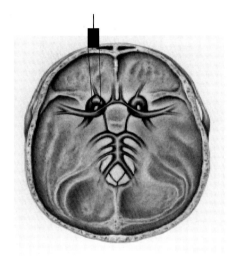

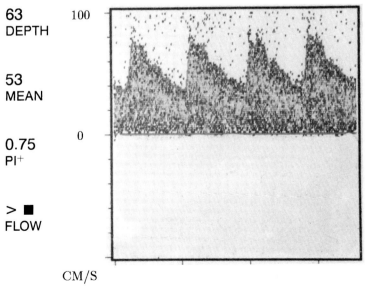

63
DEPTH

53
MEAN

0.75
PI⁺

> ■
FLOW

100

0

CM/S

Figure 5.19 Insonation of the carotid siphon.

Retro-Submandibular Window (Fig. 5.20)

The patient should be in the supine position with the head slightly extended, in order to allow the transducer to be placed properly. In turn, the transducer should rest below and behind the mandible, immediately adjacent to the angle of the mandible. In patients whose necks are very short, the head may need to be extended further.

Extracranial ICA Characteristics:

Depth   50mm
Direction   Away
Window   Retromandibular

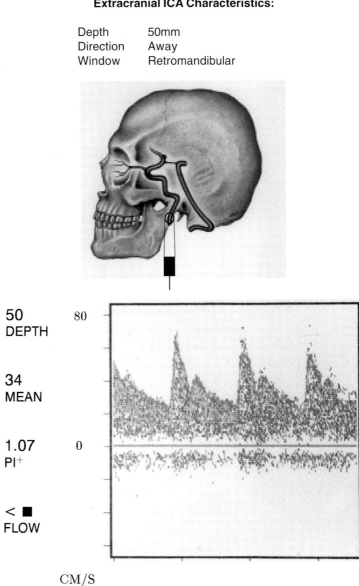

Figure 5.20 Insonation of the extracranial ICA.

The extracranial portion of the ICA can be assessed using the submandibular window. The flow direction of the vessel is away from the probe, and the Doppler waveform is obtained at a depth of 50 mm. The normal velocity is between 24 and 48 cm/s. Variations in the velocity may occur with minor changes in the probe position. This window, unlike the cranial windows, does not provide a hard surface for probe placement, but rather a soft and fleshy area, allowing great variability in probe positioning.

Care needs to be taken not to confuse the external carotid artery with the ICA. Changing the probe angle, alternatively, allows delineation of both an external carotid artery signal (high resistance and usually more medial on the neck) and an ICA signal (lower resistance and usually more lateral on the neck). A relatively large amount of ultrasonic gel may need to be used in order to ensure adequate interface between the transducer and the skin.

Pitfalls in Vessel Identification

Because imaging is not involved, the ability to assess the cerebral circulation is as much an art as it is a science. The identification of any vessel using TCD depends upon the following factors:

> window used for the examination,
> depth of the sample volume,
> flow direction in relationship to the probe,
> traceability of the vessel,
> spatial relationship with the other vessels,
> size of the skull,
> response to common carotid artery compression or vibration.

In addition, the examiner must take into account a variety of factors that contribute to potential pitfalls in TCD examination. Approximately 50% of the population have a complete Circle of Willis, whereas the other 50% have anatomic variations. The most common variations are an absent ACoA or PCoA. The ACA may also be absent, or hypoplastic, and the PCA may branch directly from the ICA (see Fig. 2.6). The most common problems encountered in TCD practice include the following.

Identifying the PCA

The PCA is often confused with the MCA because they are located in the same axial plane. However, they are at different depths along the ultrasound beam and this makes possible their differentiation. Several useful techniques include the following:

- While insonating the PCA at a depth of 65 or 70 mm, decrease the sample volume depth to 55 to 50 mm without changing the probe position. The Doppler signal should disappear at 50 or 55 mm if the signal was obtained from the PCA. But, if the Doppler signal remains constant, then most likely the recording has been from the MCA, and the probe will need to be angled more posterior and slightly inferior for PCA assessment.

- Ask the patient to close his/her eyes while insonating the PCA. It should be possible to note a decrease in the audible signal, as well as an approximate 20% decrease in velocity. Then, the patient should be asked to open his/her eyes. A few seconds later, the audible signal and the velocity should increase back to baseline measurements. The changes in velocity are due to the light-dependent change in blood flow demand by the visual cortex, commonly supplied by the Calcarine artery, a branch of the PCA.

While obtaining a velocity measurement from the PCA, usually at a depth of 65 mm, the flow direction may be toward or away from the probe, depending upon whether the P1 or the P2 segments of the vessel are insonated, respectively. The PCoA can be assessed when there is a large enough flow volume through it to produce a Doppler shift to be analyzed. Flow direction is variable, depending upon the pathology present.

Identifying the Vertebral Arteries

The vertebral arteries may be tortuous or located very close together and, therefore, difficult to identify by TCD as individual arteries. Compression of the extracranial VA against the mastoid may also assist in their identification.

Identifying a Cause of Reversed Flow Direction in the ACA

Changes in ACA velocities can be confusing, because there are possible anatomical variations. Reversal of ACA flow direction can be seen in patients with severe stenosis or occlusion of the proximal ICA. However, it is also possible to identify a reversal of ACA flow without concomitant ipsilateral carotid pathology. This can occur when an absent A1 segment is substituted by a large recurrent artery of Huebner.

Special Considerations

The most important aspect of performing a successful TCD study (in any environment) is that the patient is positioned so the technologist has easy access to the patient's head. Choose the side of the bed that offers the most accessibility to the patient's head before setting up the instrument. The siderail should be positioned down for easier access to the patient. Positioning the patient on their side for access to the vertebrobasilar arteries is especially important for accurate velocity assessment.

Postoperative patients may have incisions from craniotomies. These incisions are sometimes closed using staples, which can interfere with the transmission of ultrasound, or sutures, which may interfere with transducer placement (Fig. 5.21). Therefore, the transducer must be placed either in front of, or behind, the sutures or staples, requiring an alter-

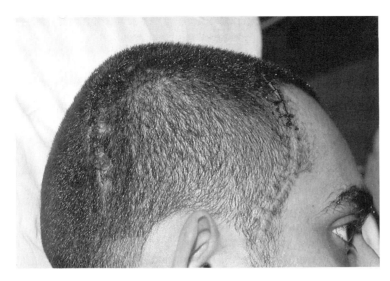

Figure 5.21 Craniotomy incision located in area of the temporal window.

ation of the plane for insonation of the vessels. The patient's head may be covered with bandages that extend over the area of the temporal window and must be cut back to perform the TCD study. Using bandage scissors, one cut in the bandage is usually all that is required to allow peeling back the bandage and exposing the temporal window (Fig. 5.22). The scalp is usually resistant to infection; therefore, sterile technique is not required. However, cleaning the area after performing the TCD study with an antiseptic swab is recommended. Swelling may occur if the patient has had surgery or a traumatic head injury, and due to this, the normal depths for insonating the vessels may need to be altered as the edema evolves.

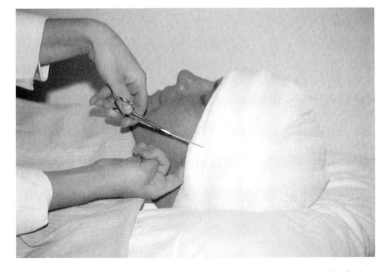

Figure 5.22 Cutting of bandage to allow exposure of temporal window.

Neurosurgical patients may be in various states of consciousness, from fully alert to comatose. These patients may act inappropriately and can be agitated or hostile. If the patient is agitated and requires sedation, this should be done before attempting the TCD study. Planning the TCD exam with the nurses may allow scheduling the study after medication has been given to help the patient relax and cooperate. Other patients may be in a constant state of motion and, therefore, obtaining a technically adequate study may be impossible.

Performing TCD Emboli Monitoring

Monitoring of potential emboli (HITS) can be performed at the patient's bedside, or in the operating room during surgical procedures (carotid endarterectomy, coronary artery bypass). The principal arteries for monitoring emboli are the MCAs through the temporal window, the cervical ICA above the angles of the jaw, and the CCA low in the neck. A 2-MHz pulsed Doppler probe is used for all three locations; however, a continuous wave Doppler may be used for the carotid arteries.

Embolic Source

Heart emboli may be detected bilaterally in any of the arteries noted above. Emboli that arise from the carotid bifurcation can be detected unilaterally in the cervical ICA and MCA. Carotid siphon emboli can be detected unilaterally in the MCA.

Embolic Rate

Embolic rate is computed as emboli per hour (EPH). Emboli monitoring should be at least 15 min (30 min desirable) on each artery of interest, even if many emboli are detected.

Calculation would be: 400 emboli over 4 h of monitoring, 400/4 = 100 EPH; 20 emboli over 15 min of monitoring, 20 × 4 = 80 EPH.

Instrumentation

Select emboli monitoring mode. Use of proper settings is critical for display, recognition, and analysis of the embolic signal. Ensure the following conditions:

proper probe fixation,
reduce gain to produce outline of spectral edge only,
use gray scale,
bidirectional display to confirm unidirectional feature of the embolus signal,
60 dB range to prevent amplitude aliasing (optimal decibel range may vary depending on the manufacturer).

Embolic Features (Fig. 5.23)

1. Unidirectional.
2. Short duration (0.1 s).
3. 6 to 60 dB above background velocity spectrum.
4. Sounds like a chirp (particulate) or a moan (air).

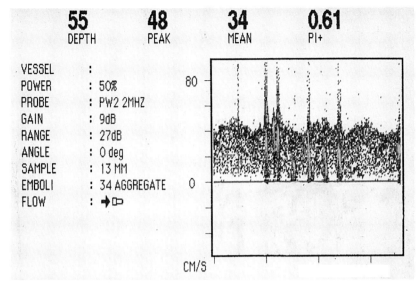

Figure 5.23 Embolic signals.

Reporting Emboli

1. Number counted per hour (EPH).
2. Decibel strength of embolic signal.
3. Location detected.

The instrument will aggregate the embolic signals throughout the monitoring time. Screens need to be saved when emboli are noted, unless a videotape recorder is used. This allows playback of the emboli signals and hard copy printing for the report.

Calculating Decibel Strength

Postprocess the signal by decreasing the gain low enough to display the emboli signal only, and note the decibel. Further decrease the gain until the emboli signal disappears and again record the decibel. The difference between the two equals the total decibel strength of the embolic signal. A variety of emboli signals may have different decibel strength, depending on the size or type and speed at which they travel through the stream of red blood cells. A range of decibel signals may be reported.

Bubble emboli may be more reflective of the ultrasound than particulate; however, due to considerable overlap, differentiating air from particulate is uncertain.

Particulate emboli may be monitored in the following patient conditions:

- carotid artery ulceration or thrombus,
- siphon stenosis,
- transient ischemic attacks and stroke,
- prosthetic valves and atrial fibrillation.

Gas or air emboli may be detected during the following procedures:

- cardiopulmonary bypass and cardiotomy procedures,
- neurosurgical procedures,
- carotid endarterectomy,
- contrast injections for cardiac septal defects.

Microemboli monitoring can be diagnostic for a site of origin of embolization and may provide a guide for therapeutic measures in the prevention of stroke.

Performing Cerebrovascular Reactivity Testing

The use of TCD in evaluating induced CO_2 vasomotor response has been defined by several investigators. The theoretical background and methods will be described.

CO_2 is a potent vasodilator; therefore, an increase in the arterial P_{CO_2} (hypercapnia) causes dilatation of the small, distal, resistant vessels in the brain. When the distal arterioles are dilated, the peripheral vascular resistance is decreased, thereby allowing an increase in the cerebral blood flow. In contrast, a reduction in the arterial P_{CO_2} (hypocapnia) causes vasoconstriction of the small, distal, resistant vessels in the brain. When the distal arterioles are constricted, the peripheral vascular resistance is increased, resulting in a decrease in cerebral blood flow. Using TCD, changes in blood flow can be indirectly measured, because CO_2 concentration does not affect the diameter of the large proximal arterial vessels. Therefore, by manipulating the concentration of P_{CO_2}, the changes in MCA velocities directly reflect changes in the diameter of the vasomotor arterioles. Assessing the cerebrovascular reserve is a method for challenging the brain's microcirculatory changes in response to changes in P_{CO_2} and it is not to be confused with autoregulation.

Prior to performing the TCD with CO_2 manipulation, the patient should be instructed completely in what can be expected during the testing period. Cooperation is enhanced when the patient understands what they will be expected to do, how long it will take, and the normal sensations they may experience. The patient should be instructed to report any symptoms that would cause discontinuance of the test, such as chest pain, numbness, tingling, or severe shortness of breath. Both the inhalation of CO_2 and hyperventilation may cause dryness of the mouth. Lightheadedness may be experienced during hyperventilation, and is entirely normal. These feelings should all subside immediately, after resuming normal breathing of room air.

The patient is placed supine on a stretcher or hospital bed and instructed to rest comfortably. Although patients may sit upright, they most often feel more relaxed in the supine position. The TCD instrument should be set up and the endtidal CO_2 analyzer properly calibrated. Depending on the equipment used, a system with either a face mask or mouthpiece with a one-way valve and nose clip should be applied to the patient for acclimation of the test procedure. The bilateral temporal windows can be assessed while the patient is resting and breathing room

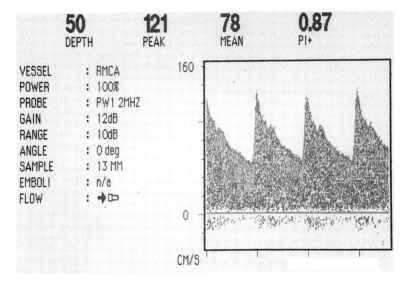

Figure 5.24 Baseline velocity of MCA.

air. A complete TCD is performed to assess the entire Circle of Willis prior to beginning the vasomotor reactivity test.

To begin the CO_2 challenge, the best signal in the bilateral MCAs, usually at a depth between 50 and 55 mm, should be obtained and baseline velocities recorded (Fig. 5.24) while also recording the baseline end tidal CO_2. The mixture of 94% oxygen and 6% CO_2 is now infused adequately through the flowmeter system (8 to 10 L/min) while continuous MCA velocities and end-tidal CO_2 measurements are recorded. The patient is instructed to breath normally during the next 3 to 5 min while the velocities should reach their maximum (Fig. 5.25), with an increase in the end tidal CO_2 to 20% above baseline measurements. Again, the

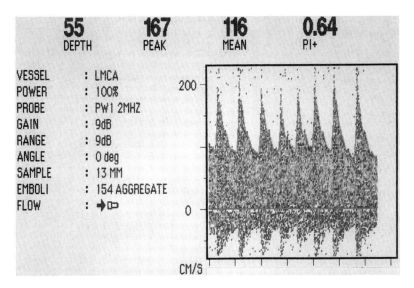

Figure 5.25 Maximum velocity obtained in MCA during inhalation of oxygen/ CO_2 mixture.

highest velocities and the accompanying end tidal CO_2 measurements are recorded, after which the flowmeter is turned off and the patient begins to breath room air.

Immediately after the velocities and end tidal CO_2 measurements return to baseline, the patient is instructed to hyperventilate. Many patients require coaching through the hyperventilation phase, for maximum effort, cooperation, and reassurance. Diligence in hyperventilation normally produces a very fast decrease in both the velocities and the end tidal CO_2 measurements. Once the velocities and the end tidal CO_2 measurements have reached their lowest, they are again recorded (Fig. 5.26). The patient is then instructed to breath normally, at which time the velocities and end tidal CO_2 measurements are recorded until they stabilize at baseline measurements. This completes the CO_2 challenge test. The patient may be offered a drink of water for complaints of dryness of mouth, and allowed to acclimate for several minutes to assure that any previous feelings of lightheadedness or dizziness have abated.

Even though the CVR testing is considered harmless, the following information should be considered. A history of severe pulmonary disease may be a contraindication for this test, as it may cause severe dyspnea. Hyperventilation has been reported to cause seizures in less than 0.5% of normal subjects. Should patients experience any discomfort that is alarming to them, the test should be aborted immediately. If respiratory, neurologic, or cardiac symptoms persist, a physician should be notified while the ultrasonographer stays with the patient.

Calculating the vasomotor reactivity has been described by Ringelstein et al. as follows. Mean flow velocity during inhalation of room air is considered 100% (baseline). This baseline measurement of mean flow velocity is compared to the percentage change in mean flow

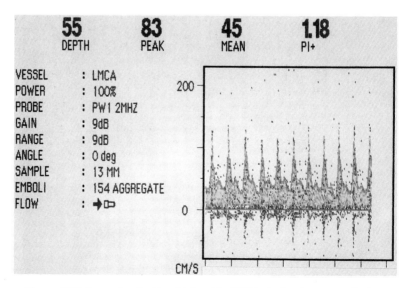

Figure 5.26 Lowest velocity obtained in MCA during hyperventilation.

velocity during inhalation of 6% CO_2 mixed with 94% oxygen (hypercapnia) and to the mean flow velocity during hyperventilation (hypocapnia) (Fig. 5.27).

$$\text{Percentage change in VMR} = \frac{V_{MCA}(\text{hypercapnia}) - V_{MCA}(\text{hypocapnia})}{V_{MCA}(\text{baseline})}$$

$$\text{Percentage change in } P_{CO_2} \text{ torr} = \frac{P_{CO_2}(\text{hypercapnia}) - P_{CO_2}(\text{hypocapnia})}{P_{CO_2}(\text{baseline})}$$

Vasomotor reactivity is categorized arbitrarily as the following:

Severe reduction	<34%
Moderate reduction	34–66%
Normal	>66%.

The vasomotor reactivity test has been utilized for assessing the intactness of the circle of Willis and the capacity of the collateral circulation to compensate for blood flow reductions due to extracranial obstructions. This information can be helpful in identifying patients who are at risk for low-flow infarctions due to inability of the brain arteries to further dilate

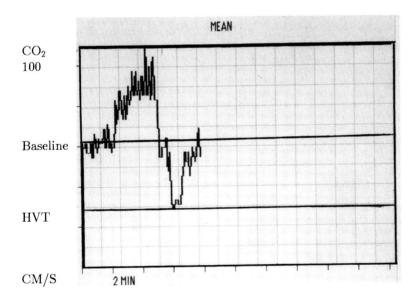

V_{MCA} Hypercapnia = 106 cm/sec
V_{MCA} Hypocapnia = 28 cm/sec
V_{MCA} Baseline = 106 cm/sec
Vasomotor Reactivity = 1.25

Figure 5.27 Graphic representation of changes in mean MCA velocities during vasomotor reactivity testing.

in response to a diminishing perfusion pressure. In contrast, the vasoconstrictive capacity of the cerebral arteries in the patients who have sustained severe head injuries may be impaired, thus not permitting hyperventilation to therapeutically decrease intracranial pressure. The greatest utility thus far in assessing vasomotor reactivity is to identify stroke-prone patients with severely reduced vasomotor reactivity, who may be asymptomatic in spite of marginal cerebral blood supply.

Selected Readings

1. Ringelstein EB, Sievers C, Ecker S., et al. Noninvasive assessment of CO_2-induced cerebral vasomotor response in normal individuals and patients with internal carotid artery occlusions. *Stroke.* 1988;19:963–969.
2. Saver J, Feldmann E. Basic TCD examination: technique and anatomy, In *Transcranial Doppler ultrasonography*, Babikian VL, Wecksler LR (eds). St. Louis: C.V. Mosby; 1993:16–17.
3. Spencer MP. Detection of cerebral arterial emboli, In *Transcranial Doppler*, Newell DW, Aaslid R (eds). New York: Raven Press; 1992:215–230.

Principles and Strategies for TCD Interpretation

Once the transcranial Doppler (TCD) data have been acquired, the clinician faces the challenge of interpreting the study, and deciding whether or not the findings are normal. Furthermore, if the TCD is abnormal, the interpreter will also be required to express an opinion regarding the clinical significance of the abnormality. The interpretation should be sufficiently informative to be relevant and helpful to the referring physician, otherwise the purpose of performing TCD will be questioned from that point on. A common problem encountered in daily practice is the inappropriate referral of patients for TCD examination, in search of answers to questions that TCD is not capable of addressing. For example, as it is stated throughout this book, TCD is a very useful tool in the detection and follow-up of vasospasm following aneurysmal subarachnoid hemorrhage. However, it is practically impossible to perform a TCD in the expectation of detecting the aneurysm itself. Therefore, to be clinically useful, TCD must only be used to search for conditions that it is capable of detecting. In addition to this, we also feel that certain other prerequisites are necessary in order to provide day-to-day quality interpretation of TCD studies.

Prerequisites

The interpretation of TCD is somewhat different than that of extracranial vascular ultrasound studies. The principal difference is that the vessels accessible by TCD (all 13 of them!) are interconnected anatomically and, therefore, hemodynamic changes in any one of them will have significant repercussions upon the rest. In order to assure that the interpretation of TCD studies is of high quality, the following prerequisites are recommended.

Technically Adequate Data

As with any other diagnostic technique, the quality of TCD data is operator dependent. The performance of TCD studies by trained and qualified sonographers will assist the interpreter in assuring that the data are of high quality, that the Doppler waveforms have been appropriately sampled, and that the possibility of technical error has been minimized. Quality assurance of the technical data is best accomplished by a close collaboration between the sonographer and the interpreter. In order to translate this collaboration into a quality assurance process, we recommend for sonographers to be required to provide independent intramural (within the laboratory) interpretation of the tests. This can be internally compared with that provided by the clinician in order to detect discrepancies and misunderstandings that could potentially lead to on-going errors in data acquisition. Along these lines, we also recommend that the sonographers and the clinicians have joint sessions of interpretation as often as possible (no less than once per week). In our experience, this is probably one of the most difficult things to accomplish, but it is also one of the most rewarding, particularly when training new technologists. Finally, in our opinion, it is of utmost importance for the clinician to be conversant with the performance of TCD studies. It is only by having experience in the acquisition of TCD data that one can optimally estimate the problems that may be encountered during the interpretation process.

Systematic Approach

Once the data are available for interpretation, the approach to the information should be systematic. The steps described below should be followed persistently and consistently for every study being interpreted. This will assure that every possible variable (of which there are plenty) is considered when reaching a diagnostic impression. Interpreting TCD studies is as much an art as it is a science, and it is most comparable to the interpretation of electroencephalograms. The Doppler waveforms from up to 13 vessels are considered both independently and in group, while attempting to identify abnormal patterns. In addition, we strongly recommend consideration of the TCD data concurrently with the information obtained by means of extracranial duplex (or color Doppler imaging) ultrasound.

Quality Control Process

Every laboratory must have a quality control process that will allow critical review of the TCD data. This process should emphasize review of other diagnostic studies (e.g., angiography) on a regular basis, and feedback to the sonographers about discrepancies found, as well as their possible explanation. In addition, there is no substitute for experience and, therefore, cases that deviate from the routine should be archived in teaching files and the findings used as a resource of information for future reference.

Parameters for Interpretation

The most important variables measured by TCD are blood flow velocities: mean (V_m), peak systolic (V_{ps}), and end diastolic (V_{ed}). Normal values for all these velocities have been published, and those reported for V_m (in the context of specific criteria for vessel identification, which include depth of sampling and direction of flow) are summarized in Table 5.1. In addition, another parameter that must be taken into account is the pulsatility index (PI). There are several formulas currently in use for its calculation. The one most commonly utilized is that proposed by Gosling: $PI = V_{ps} - V_{ed}/V_m$. Its normal range approximates 0.85 to 1.10, but it is important to clarify that the PI should be utilized more as a qualitative parameter than a quantitative one. Pulsatility is a concept that relates systolic and diastolic measurements: the greater the difference between the two, the greater the pulsatility. However, the PI is a parameter that can be affected by many variables, the most important of which are distal resistance to flow (either intracranial pressure or vascular constriction), systemic blood pressure, cardiac function, and even proximal vascular pathology. As it is currently understood, the PI is probably a misnomer because there is evidence that its value does not correlate with the actual arterial pulsatility. Therefore, one must be careful with its use during interpretation. In our experience, the PI is helpful as an adjunct criterion to assess changes in resistance to flow in specific areas of the cerebral circulation.

The Interpretation Process

The two objectives of TCD interpretation are: a) the recognition of abnormal patterns, and b) their integration into a clinically correlative diagnosis (allowing for differential diagnosis). The first objective is somewhat of a prerequisite for the second, because having found a "normal" TCD pattern will effectively end the interpretation of that particular study. In order to minimize the chances of error during the interpretation of TCD studies, we recommend that the following sequential steps are taken for every study interpreted.

Single Vessel Assessment

The first step in the interpretation of TCD studies is the assessment of every vessel that was studied. In order to decide whether each vessel shows normal or abnormal hemodynamics, a critical examination of the parameters mentioned must be conducted. Under normal circumstances, the velocities measured in the cerebral arteries must fall within the normal range (which we consider to be two standard deviations from the mean value), and there should not be significant side-to-side differences between homologous vessels. In general, the V_m is the most important velocity to measure, whereas the V_{ps} and V_{ed} are reviewed in the context of pulsatility assessment (see below). From the concepts outlined, the velocities measured (if not normal) can either be abnormally increased or abnormally decreased.

It is very important for the clinician interpreting TCD studies to understand that the test does not provide a measure of cerebral blood flow, but of blood flow velocities. Along these lines, it must also be understood that: $CBF = CBFV \times LA$, where CBF is the cerebral blood flow, CBFV is the cerebral blood flow velocity, and LA is the luminal area. Based upon this formula, it is easy to derive that a 30% reduction in the diameter of the vessel being examined will result in doubling (two times) of the measured V_m. This is a very important concept, for it underscores the sensitivity of TCD to changes in vessel diameter, which may not be detectable by other neuroimaging techniques such as angiography. An important point to repeat is that, if the clinician finds all individual vessels to have normal hemodynamic characteristics, he needs to go no further, the TCD study is automatically interpreted as normal. If, on the other hand, some abnormalities are found, the steps that follow must be taken.

Pattern Recognition

After having decided that one or more of the vessels that were individually examined show some type of an abnormality, the clinician must determine the distribution of these abnormalities (Table 6.1). This allows him to construct a differential diagnosis of all reasonable explanations for the abnormal hemodynamic pattern. It is possible to predict the various hemodynamic patterns that can be encountered in practice based upon considering velocity abnormalities and their possible distributions (Table 6.1). In general, abnormal velocities can be either too high or too low, and their distribution can be in all vessels, a single vessel, or a group of vessels. In addition, in many instances it will be necessary to consider associated findings related to other parameters (e.g., PI) in the identification of the abnormal pattern present. The ability to recognize patterns of TCD abnormality directly relates to experience, for which there is no substitute. Nevertheless, it is possible to increase the effectiveness of

Table 6.1 Different hemodynamic patterns that can be recognized when interpreting TCD.

Pattern	Example
Abnormally high V_m	
Single vessel	atheromatous stenosis; vasospasm
All vessels	anemia
Group of vessels	arteriovenous malformation; vasospasm
Abnormally low V_m	
Single vessel	upstream flow-reducing lesion
All vessels	poor cardiac function; coma states
Groups of vessels	upstream occlusion
Abnormally high PI	
Single vessel	downstream occlusion
All vessels	Increased ICP
Abnormally low PI	
Single vessel	upstream flow-reducing lesion
Group of vessels	arteriovenous malformation

V_m = mean blood flow velocity, PI = pulsatility index, ICP = intracranial pressure.

one's interpretative skills by simply keeping in mind that the findings in all vessels sampled must "make sense," that is, they must correlate and have a logical interrelation. Every TCD diagnostic proposition must be tested according to this principle. If some part of the TCD study does not "fit" with the proposed abnormal pattern, an error or a variant must be sought.

Doppler Waveform Analysis

The assessment of Doppler waveforms obtained by TCD is more complex than that which is performed in extracranial vascular ultrasound, and it has not been as exploited in the past. In addition to blood flow velocities, other parameters such as PI and abnormal flow direction must be also utilized when making the final analysis of the data reviewed. Pulsatility indices provide the interpreter with information about the distal resistance of the cerebral vasculature. As noted previously, however, this information is more qualitative than quantitative, and we caution new TCD adepts about developing too close of an attachment to the values of any of these indices. In general, the TCD Doppler waveform can be said to be more or less pulsatile than it is expected or found in other vessels in the same patient. Furthermore, the slope of the systolic upstroke can provide information about cardiac output and proximal flow-reducing lesions. Doppler spectral widening, however, is not generally applicable to TCD because of the spatial relationship between the vessel and the Doppler sample volume.

The TCD Report

After the clinician has finished interpreting the TCD data, a report must be generated. In general, we recommend caution when reporting TCD findings. The interpretation of TCD studies should lead first to a hemodynamic diagnosis, and second to a clinical correlation diagnosis. A common pitfall is that of "reading into" the TCD studies. This occurs when the clinician who is interpreting the study is also the referring physician and, during interpretation, he uses knowledge acquired at the bedside to "steer" the TCD interpretation and make it fit the clinical scenario. We strongly advise against the temptation of entering external variables into the interpretation process in this fashion. The TCD findings should stand by themselves, and the finding of a specific abnormal hemodynamic pattern should always lead to the same type of report, including a differential diagnosis of all processes capable of giving rise to such a pattern.

Special Situations

Monitoring

Reporting the results of TCD monitoring requires, in addition to what has been said, the ability to recognize and interpret trends, as well as changes that take place along them. In addition, our practice has been to report the concurrent values of non-TCD data simultaneously acquired, such as heart rate, blood pressure, intracranial pressure, among others. In general, this requires the utilization of special reporting forms that provide referring physicians with a table displaying the changes noted.

Emboli Detection

The detection of emboli and its interpretation requires some basic understanding of cerebrovascular anatomy and physiology. The salient features that relate to this are: location and origin, and rate and strength of the high intensity transients (HITs). Cardiac and aortic emboli may be detected in any of the cerebral arteries, although they may show a preference to be found in the middle cerebral arteries (MCAs). Emboli that arise from common carotid artery (CCA) bifurcation plaques are usually detected ipsilaterally in the cervical or intracranial internal carotid artery (ICA), or its branches (anterior and middle cerebral arteries). It is important to emphasize that, in 20% (one in five) of the general population, the posterior cerebral artery (PCA) retains a persistent fetal circulatory pattern and its flow derives from the ipsilateral ICA rather than from the basilar artery (BA). Emboli that originate in the vertebral arteries (VA) are usually detected in the BA or the PCAs.

The embolic rate is reported as emboli per hour (EPH) and it should be adjusted to reflect a prediction derived from the actual monitoring period. For example, 400 emboli found during a 4-h period of monitoring results in $400/4 = 100$ EPH, and, conversely, 20 emboli found during 15 min results in $20 \times 4 = 80$ EPH.

Some TCD instruments will aggregate the HITs throughout the monitoring time. This usually requires that screens are saved when emboli are noted. An alternative, less efficient method is that of saving the studies using standard videotapes so they can be counted later.

In order to report the strength of the HITs, the decibels of the background TCD waveform must be subtracted. Once this is done, as described elsewhere in the book, the clinician can report a range of decibels for the HITs found. In general, air emboli are said to have higher impedance and higher decibels than formed emboli. However, at the time of this writing, the differentiation between these is not reliable.

Cerebrovascular Reserve Capacity

In specific cases, cerebral vasomotor reactivity (VMR) can be assessed by challenging the cerebral circulation under conditions of changes in partial pressure of CO_2. The methodology has been described elsewhere in the book, and we will only deal with its interpretation. Because the most important indication for assessing cerebral VMR is to determine the cerebrovascular reserve capacity, the important finding would be a reduction of cerebral VMR. This is calculated by assigning the V_m during room air breathing a baseline value of 100%, and comparing it to the percentage change during hyperventilation (hypocapnia) and during 6% CO_2 inhalation (hypercapnia), as follows:

$$\%\Delta VMR = \frac{V_m(\text{hypercapnia}) - V_m(\text{hypocapnia})}{V_m(\text{baseline})}.$$

The cerebrovascular reserve capacity is considered to be impaired when the cerebral VMR is reduced. The existing criteria are such that a VMR <34% indicates a significant impairment of cerebrovascular reserve capacity. In turn, VMR >66% is considered normal, and values between 34 and 66% are equivocal. As noted previously, its most important usefulness is to detect significant hemodynamic impairment of the brain circulation, and individuals at risk for ischemia.

Selected Readings

1. Aaslid R, Markwalder TM, Nornes H. Noninvasive transcranial Doppler ultrasound recording of flow velocity in basal cerebral arteries. *J. Neurosurg.* 1982;57:769–774.
2. Arnolds BJ, von Reutern GM. Transcranial Doppler sonography. Examination technique and normal reference values. *Ultrasound Med Biol.* 1986; 12:115–123.
3. DeWitt LD, Rosengart A, Teal P. Transcranial Doppler sonography: normal values. In *Transrcanial Doppler sonography*, Babikian VL, Wechsler LR (eds). St. Louis: Mosby YearBook; 1993:29–38.
4. Ringelstein EB, et al. Npn-invasive assessment of CO_2-induced cerebral vasomotor response in normal individuals and patients with internal carotid artery occlusions. *Stroke.* 1988;19:963–969.
5. Ringelstein EB, et al. Transcranial Doppler sonograpphy: anatomical landmarks and normal velocity values. *Ultrasound Med Biol.* 1990;16:745–761.

Case Studies

The following represent a series of case studies that are illustrative of some of the major applications of TCD. They are not meant to be exclusive but simply to demonstrate the typical findings in patients with these pathologic conditions.

Example Case Study 1. Vertebral Atherosclerosis

Patient: R.W.
Age: 69 years
Gender: Man
Reason for referral: Possible vertebrobasilar insufficiency
TCD findings: Abnormally elevated mean blood flow velocities in both vertebral arteries (RVA = 136 cm/s and LVA = 132 cm/s). Basilar artery mean velocities in the upper limit of normal (58–66 cm/s). Findings are consistent with bilateral vertebral artery stenosis (Fig. 6.1).
Additional comments: Angiography demonstrated bilateral stenoses of the vertebral arteries. A single focal narrowing in the RVA and two tandem narrowings in the LVA (Fig. 6.2).

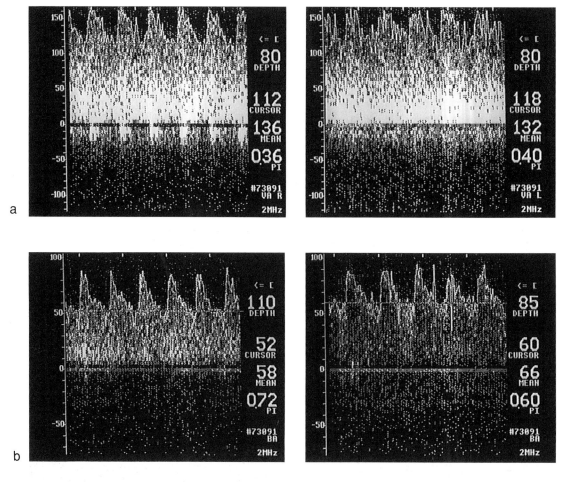

Figure 6.1 TCD waveforms of both vertebral arteries (a), and of the basilar artery (b). The Vm are as follows RVA 5 136 cm/sec, LVA 5 132 cm/sec, and BA 5 58-66 cm/sec.

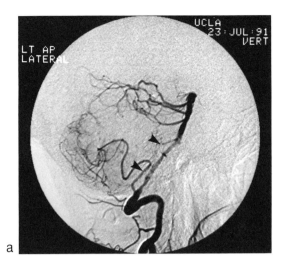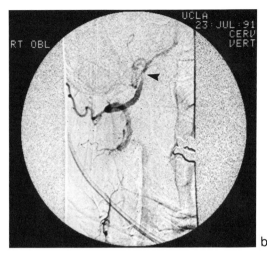

a   b

Figure 6.2 Angiographic images of the LVA (a) and RVA (b) injections demonstrating the segmental stenosis of these vessels (arrows).

Example Case Study 2. Middle Cerebral Artery Atherosclerosis

Patient: C.L.
Age: 41 years
Gender: Woman
Reason for referral: Left hemiparesis
TCD findings: Abnormally elevated mean blood flow velocities in the right middle cerebral artery (RMCA = 120 cm/s), in comparison with normal velocities in the contralateral vessel (Fig. 6.3).
Additional comments: Although the patient had a questionable history of migraine, the TCD findings are highly suggestive of RMCA atherosclerotic narrowing.

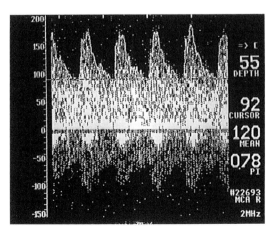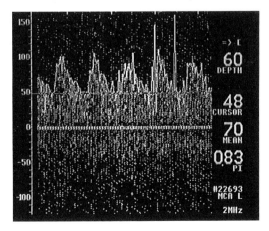

a   b

Figure 6.3 Side-to-side differences in the Vm of the middle cerebral arteries. The RMCA 120 cm/sec, while the LMCA 70 cm/sec.

Example Case Study 3. Cerebral Vasospasm and Follow-up

Patient: E.W.

Age: 36 years

Gender: Woman

Reason for referral: Subarachnoid hemorrhage 10 days earlier

TCD findings: Abnormally elevated mean blood flow velocities in both middle cerebral arteries (RMCA = 205 cm/s and LMCA = 232 cm/s) consistent with severe vasospasm. In addition, the proximal internal carotid arteries showed relatively normal velocities, resulting in elevated velocity ratios [V_m (MCA/ICA) >4] (Fig. 6.4).

Additional comments: Angiography demonstrates spasm of the terminal ICA and MCA origin (Fig. 6.5). The findings improve following angioplasty.

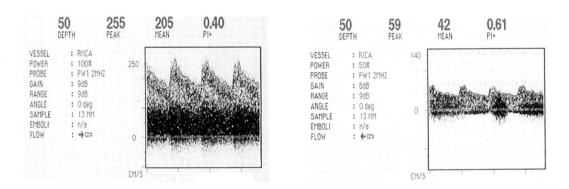

Figure 6.4 TCD waveforms of the RMCA and proximal RICA, showing significant differences in Vm, suggestive of intracranial vasospasm.

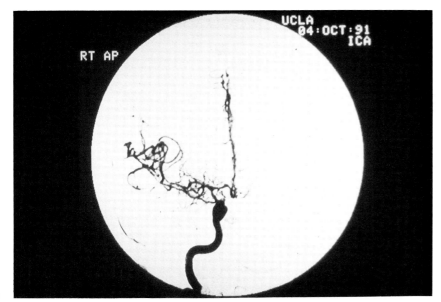

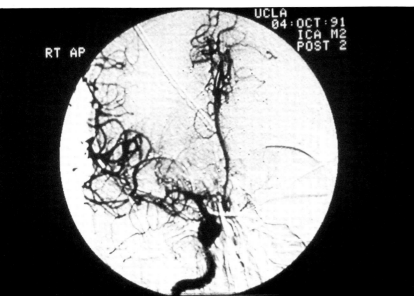

Figure 6.5 (a) Angiography demonstrates spasm of the terminal RICA at the RMCA origin. (b) Angiography following angioplasty reveals improvement.

Example Case Study 4. Arteriovenous Malformation

Patient: M.B.
Age: 32 years
Gender: Man
Reason for referral: Arteriovenous malformation
TCD findings: Abnormally elevated mean blood flow velocities in the left middle cerebral artery (LMCA = 170 cm/s) with relatively decreased pulsatility (PI = 0.46) are suggestive of an AVM-feeding artery. In comparison, the ipsilateral ICA velocity is slightly elevated, resulting in decreased velocity ratios [V_m (MCA/ICA) <3] (Fig. 6.6).
Additional comments: Angiography shows a moderate-size AVM being fed by the LMCA (Fig. 6.7). Embolization is followed by obliteration of the malformation and normalization of TCD findings.

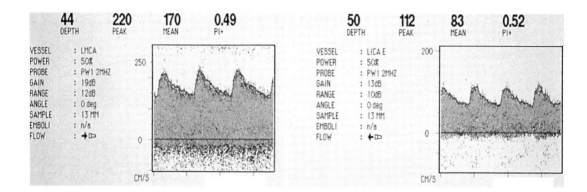

Figure 6.6 TCD waveforms of the LMCA showing elevated velocities (Vm 170 cm/sec) and reduced pulsatility (PI 0.49), The LICA velocities are only minimally increased (Vm 83 cm/sec).

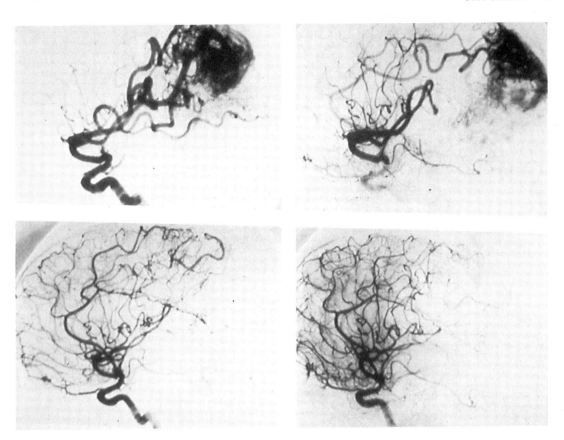

Figure 6.7 Angiography shows the AVM as it is fed by the LMCA, and its obliteration by embolization.

Example Case Study 5. Brain Death

Patient: S.W.

Age: 29 years

Gender: Man

Reason for referral: Severe head injury

TCD findings: Immediate TCD findings did not show any significant abnormalities. As intracranial pressure increased, and cerebral perfusion pressure decreased, the patient's condition deteriorated. One day later, the patient met clinical criteria for brain death, and the TCD findings were consistent with cerebral circulatory arrest (Fig. 6.8).

Additional comments: The hemodynamic changes leading to brain death are progressive and not instantaneous. Therefore, TCD studies must be repeated several times along the course of the patient's hospitalization.

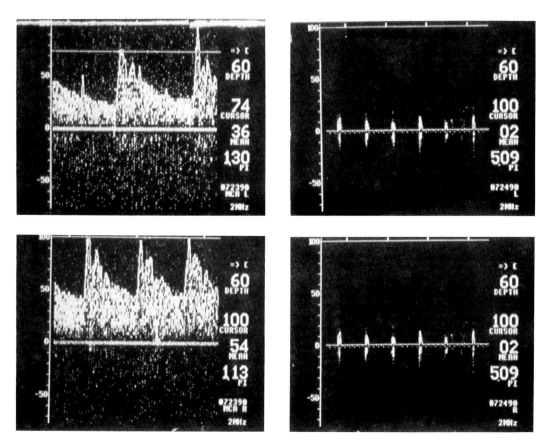

Figure 6.8 The immediate TCD findings shows normal appearing waveforms (left). One day later, the findings are consistent with circulatory arrest (right).

Index

Index